End Emotional Outsourcing

How to Overcome Your Codependent, Perfectionist, and People-Pleasing Habits

BEATRIZ VICTORIA ALBINA

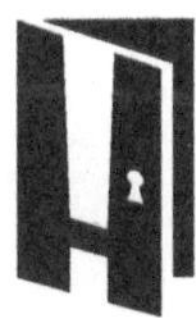

Cover design by Jim Datz. Cover photo by Shutterstock.

First published in the US in 2025 by Balance,
an imprint of Grand Central Publishing
The Balance name and logo are registered trademarks
of Hachette Book Group, Inc

First published in the UK in 2025 by Headline Home
An imprint of Headline Publishing Group Limited

2

Cataloguing in Publication Data is available from the British Library

Trade Paperback ISBN 978 1 0354 1473 4
ebook ISBN 978 1 0354 1474 1

Offset in 11.96/16.12pt Dante MT Pro by Six Red Marbles UK, Thetford, Norfolk

Printed and bound in Great Britain by Clays Ltd, Elcograf S.p.A.

Headline's policy is to use papers that are natural, renewable and recyclable products and made from wood grown in well-managed forests and other controlled sources. The logging and manufacturing processes are expected to conform to the environmental regulations of the country of origin.

Headline Publishing Group Limited
An Hachette UK Company
Carmelite House
50 Victoria Embankment
London EC4Y 0DZ

The authorised representative in the EEA is Hachette Ireland,
8 Castlecourt Centre, Dublin 15, D15 XTP3, Ireland (email: info@hbgi.ie)

www.headline.co.uk
www.hachette.co.uk

To my wife, Billey Albina—who embodies the kind of love that is both liberatory and deeply generative, ever-expanding and endlessly true. You show me, every day, what true interdependent relating feels like. Your love is my greatest homecoming.

Contents

End Emotional Outsourcing

Introduction

Are You Ready to Stop Putting Yourself Last?

My love, when was the last time you felt like you really mattered in your own life?

When was the last time your needs came first—or you even acknowledged that you had any? When was the last time you felt like you were enough or basically good, as a human? The last time you did something because you wanted to, not because you felt like you had to? How about the last time you knew what you wanted for dinner (without checking on whatever everyone else wanted first or couching your idea in "I mean, but only if you want that too, because if not we can have something else").

Can you even remember?

If you're anything like the thousands of women I've worked with, I'm willing to bet that you don't like your answer. Every day I speak with women who are sick of the constant striving to please, the expectation to be the reliable one, the never-lets-anyone-down superstar whose house is always magically spotless and who never complains. Or they're the other extreme and can't seem to get it up to actually take care of themselves and their own lives, so exhausted from performing perfection in every other area of life. For more than two decades, I have worked with women who feel lost, burned out, emotionally exhausted, or numb. They're mean to themselves and are constantly wiped out, are coping with chronic pain and gut issues, sick to death of their partner's weaponized incompetence or the dance of dating people who never quite seem to leave enough space for them, who never feel like the Right Fit, but they can't seem to leave the relationships, 'cause, well, they're in it now! They're drained by caregiving expectations, unsure of how to set boundaries and definitely not able to uphold them, sick and tired of martyring themselves, playing superwoman, and maintaining their reputation as the consummate Good Girl. They have spent their whole lives taking care of everyone except themselves. They know they can't live this way one more minute but also can't imagine another way to be.

I know this story well because I've been there myself. For as long as I can remember, I believed my value was tied to what I could do for others, and I did everything I could to not rock the boat, to keep everyone happy with me and conflict far from my life. It wasn't conscious at first—just a way of moving through the world that seemed to make sense. If I could anticipate everyone's needs, smooth things over, take responsibility for other people's feelings, and be the funny-bunny who kept folks laughing when tensions rose, then maybe I'd feel secure, loved, and worthy. So I became the caretaker, the problem solver, the jester, the mom of any and every group, and the one who had it all together on the surface.

Beneath that polished exterior, I was exhausted, disconnected from myself, and increasingly burned out. The more I tried to manage the world around me, the less control I actually felt. I was terrified that if I stopped being "useful," people would leave and I'd be alone. My sense of worth had become completely outsourced—tied to how well I could serve others, personally and professionally. It wasn't sustainable, but I didn't know any other way to live.

The tipping point came when I started to see the toll it was taking on my body. Years of putting everyone else first had left me depleted—emotionally, mentally, and physically. I struggled with chronic stress, wicked digestive issues, and a constant undercurrent of what's clinically referred to as "ughhhhhhh." My nervous system was stuck in overdrive, bracing for the next crisis to manage, always on the go-go-go, while also keeping me frozen to my feelings—the emotional gas tank long since drained. But as much as I hated my life, I had no idea how to change it all.

What began as a desire to "fix" myself—through endless books, podcasts, and therapies—slowly turned into something deeper. Always a science, biology, and psychology nerd, I started exploring somatic, or body-based, work, nervous system regulation, breathwork, and the layers of emotional patterns that kept me stuck in these cycles. Through this process, I learned to listen to my body for the first time in years. Not just to manage stress or to stop being sad, but to hear what it had been trying to tell me all along: that I was more than what I did for others. That my worth wasn't something I had to earn.

"Emotional Outsourcing" is the term I coined (and trademarked going back to when I first started using it with clients in January 2012) to describe the mind-body survival habit of chronically sourcing our sense of self-worth, safety, significance, and emotional wellness from everyone and everything outside ourselves to our own detriment, instead of believing in our own being that we are inherently worthy of love and care exactly as we are. It's the foundation for our codependent, people-pleasing, and perfectionist habits and the reason we come to believe that we have to earn love, care, and attention—that we aren't inherently worthy of it just because we exist.

Ultimately, Emotional Outsourcing is how we end up revved up, numbed out, and juggling everything—work, relationships, home—feeling that no matter how much we do, it's just never enough. It's how we end up nodding along to a dinner plan we're not excited about, or an opinion we disagree with, just because we don't want to rock the boat. It's the reason we agree to a project deadline that's humanly impossible, because we can't bear the thought of letting someone down. It's how we end up writing and rewriting every text message, worried that any slight miscommunication will lead to judgment and conflict. It's how we end up living at a crossroads where our intuition is whispering (or maybe shouting) what we need, but instead of following that inner guide, we look to a parent, partner, friend, neighbor, colleague, or maybe just the powers that be for decisions about our own lives.

So many of us, especially those of us socialized as women, have been systematically disempowered and belittled our whole lives. The systems that shaped you—your caregivers and family system, yes, but equally the oppressive systems of patriarchy, white-settler colonialism, and capitalism—led you to doubt your lovability. They taught you to hide parts of yourself away in case they were "too much." They taught you that making other people happy was more important than your own physical and emotional well-being and definitely your happiness, which comes last, for sure. They taught you that your worth is tied to how much you produce, how much you do for others, and how "successful" your life looks on paper—not how much joy, peace, ease, and beauty you live in, not how free your spirit feels, how present and intentional you are, how connected you are to your own body and desires.

By the time we're adults, we've internalized these stories that we're meant to give but not ask for more, to allow others to treat us poorly or in ways that don't really work for us, to take care of the whole world first without first taking care of ourselves, and to do it with a smile. These codependent, perfectionist, people-pleasing patterns are exhausting, but more than that, they are profoundly damaging to our minds, bodies, and relationships.

You came by these Emotional Outsourcing habits rightly, *mi amor.* Most of the women I know feel alone with this struggle. I know I did. We're stuck; we're ashamed; we don't know what's "wrong" with us... but whatever it is, we need to figure out how to fix it, *and fast*. But, my darling, let me be clear: Emotional Outsourcing isn't a personal failure. It's actually

- a set of common codependent, people-pleasing, and perfectionist thought habits;
- part and parcel of living under patriarchal, white-settler colonialist, capitalist systems of oppression;
- a bodily experience written into our tissues and nervous system; and
- a set of survival skills we learned from our family blueprint, socialization, and conditioning, not our identity.

When we are stuck in Emotional Outsourcing, we lose touch with our authenticity and our dignity. We lose track of the ways that we are beautiful, whole, autonomous beings deserving of love, care, attention, and belonging exactly as we are. These habits force us to create relationships that feel lopsided. You're the Good Girl, Mother's Little Helper, the overachiever, the fixer, superwoman, giving from an empty cup until it hurts, convinced that you have to earn love, rest, and relational safety. The more we emotionally outsource—seeking advice, validation, and answers from those around us rather than our own inner voice—the more we put our own lives and needs on hold, resenting the people we care most about while doing the most to try to make ourselves good enough to deserve their respect, attention, and love.

What if I told you that there's a way off that carousel?

When you're in the thick of codependent patterns, it can feel really hard to imagine life any other way. I know—I've been there too. You feel stuck and trapped in a life that doesn't feel like your own and like you're just gonna have to live like this forever, like there's nothing you can do to make it better, especially if you believe that living this way is who you are. Changing our whole lives starts with seeing that your codependent, people-pleasing, perfectionist habits are all survival skills you learned that are no longer serving you—they aren't who you ARE at your core.

You can retrain this.

You can rewire this.

You can rewrite and reimagine this.

And I'm going to show you how.

Through my coaching work and celebrated podcast, *Feminist Wellness*, I've helped thousands of women who've suffered from the same emotional and physical stagnation that I've felt reclaim their authenticity and their relationships.

As a family nurse practitioner trained at the University of California, San Francisco, master certified life coach, and former hospice nurse with a master's in public health, I've been board-certified by the American Academy of Nurse Practitioners and trained by Peter Levine's Somatic Experiencing Institute. I've gone deep in my studies of human psychology, behavior change and wellness, the Western medical system and alternatives, science of most every flavor, herbal medicine and my ancestral ways, holistic and mainstream nutrition, meditation, Buddhism, and psychology, and, yes, I was a slam poet in the nineties, thanks for asking. As a result, I know that our minds, bodies, and relationships all contribute to our well-being—an ethos that informs my life, my coaching, and what you'll find in this book. My love, we cannot end Emotional Outsourcing just by thinking about our habits or blaming our caregivers: To achieve lasting change, we must work with our bodies as well as our minds to rewrite our familiar patterns into ones that serve us better. Science-backed, evidence-based tools only, my love—no bootstrappin' or snake oil, no #PositiveVibesOnly, #HappyThoughtsMakeItTrue BS here.

Just as important, I know that the work of healing Emotional Outsourcing is radical and community-focused work. My intersectional feminist approach to life and health means we're going to explore the ways that our codependent, people-pleasing, perfectionist habits are the natural and expectable result of living under patriarchal, white-settler colonialist, late-stage capitalist systems of oppression—extractive systems that reinforce the narratives that our value is not inherent, that we are worthy of dignity only when we are productive, "perfect," and offer something of value to the people around us (who matter more than us and our Being).

A Note on My Social Location

I am a white Latina immigrant from occupied Mapuche land also known as Mar del Plata, Argentina, the eldest daughter and long-time mom to my little sister, raised in Providence, Rhode Island (the land of the Wôpanâak, Pauquunaukit, and Nahaganset tribes), though after a decade living and working on unceded Lenape land, more commonly known as New York City, that's the place that really feels like home. I am a queer cis femme woman married to a queer cis butch woman (and you're right if you guessed that my family doesn't really get it or approve). I am blessed with a neuro-magical ADHD brain and live with chronic illness and chronic pain. My parents have college degrees from the free Argentine public education system. I hold a bachelor's from Oberlin and master's degrees from Boston University and the University of California, San Francisco. I am currently a self-employed massive nerd with immense educational privilege—a gift that I don't take lightly.

I share all this with you, my lovely reader, because perspectives are influenced by life experiences and opportunities. As an author, it is my intention to be as inclusive and mindful as possible, and I need and want to acknowledge the perspectives I'm writing from so that you can understand the influences that shape my work.

Also, while I believe that this book can help anyone of any gender, I'm focusing on speaking to women and folks socialized as women because it's the experience I can speak to with the most authority and experience as a woman and a human assigned female at birth who has spent my life working with women.* This is not to imply that I believe in a universal experience of girlhood or womanhood, nor is it at all to say that humans of all genders don't struggle with Emotional Outsourcing (they certainly do!), but rather it is an acknowledgment of the prevalence of Emotional Outsourcing for women and of my own expertise—both personally and professionally.

No matter how it feels right now, I want you to know that in my professional opinion, the fact that you picked up and are reading this book means that you are not permaeffed, my love. While the patterns your wise mind and body adopted to survive no longer serve you, I know that you don't have to live this way forever. Our minds and bodies are remarkably resilient and have a great capacity to heal when we have the right tools and the right guidance to support them.

In part 1, we're going to explore the origins and impact of your Emotional Outsourcing survival skills. We'll look at how our families of origin and our society more broadly taught us to look outside of ourselves, to overfunction for the benefit of the people and

* I will be using the terms "women" and "girls" throughout this book to refer equally to humans socialized as women and those living as women. All women are women. Period. #notaTERF

systems around us, and to do so at our own expense. We'll look at the toll Emotional Outsourcing takes on our nervous systems and why those codependent, perfectionist, and people-pleasing habits are so persistent and pernicious in our lives. We'll also look at something called *the self-abandonment cycle*, digging into the ways your shame, self-doubt, and inner critic work together to keep you disconnected from your authentic feelings and stuck in relationship patterns that do not serve you.

Then, in part 2, I'll teach you the same tools I've used to help thousands of women make lasting changes in their lives and relationships and create a more balanced, fulfilling, and healthier way of being. You'll learn to manage your own mind and self-talk with compassion; to support your nervous system and widen your emotional capacity with somatic practices; to create a new script to rewire your habitual codependent, people-pleasing, and perfectionist thought habits; and, step-by-step, to honor your limits with boundaries.

I recommend that you keep a journal handy to support you as you read. Your journal can be digital or analog—whichever helps you to feel you have a safe, private, judgment- and distraction-free space to reflect on your experiences. You'll find journal prompts at the end of each chapter to help you go deeper, and I invite you to pause often throughout each chapter to observe your feelings, notice the physical sensations in your body, and reflect on any stories that are coming up for you. (And if you don't know what any of that means just yet, fear not! We're going to learn together.)

As you move through this book and begin to unwind your Emotional Outsourcing habits, I want you to keep in mind that healing is a process and it's not at all linear. What was built over decades doesn't heal in a day, and having a bad day doesn't mean your healing is ruined, it means you're right on track. It takes time to rewire a mind, to rebalance a stressed nervous system, and to create new relationship patterns. It takes patient persistence to foster a sense of self-worth that is not contingent on others. Rolling with the perfectionist fantasy that *poof!* you'll be "all fixed" and "totally healed" once you've finished your first read will only keep you stuck. The work of healing Emotional Outsourcing is long-haul kind of deep work because those habits are written into every part of us. Our psyche, nervous system, relationship patterns, careers—they're all wrapped up in this story that we are unworthy of love, care, safety, and connection unless and until we earn it. I promise, the changes will come when you're ready.

Don't Go It Alone

My sweet one, my perfect tender ravioli, we cannot and do not do this healing work alone. We heal so that we can be in community; we are in community so that we can heal. I invite you to share with a friend or reach out to a mental health professional, such as a therapist or a well-trained coach, that you're embarking on this journey. Ask for their support as you try new things; ask for them to hold space while you explore the places that feel hurt and stuck. You can always join us at www.beatrizalbina.com and on Instagram @beatrizvictoriaalbinanp, where you'll find a community of women and other humans just like you doing this work.

It's hard—and I might argue impossible—to change your life without the love and care of those around you. Don't shortchange yourself by trying to go it alone.

My perfect buttercup, I want to be real with you: You deserve better. I know it can feel hard to admit, but the fact that you are holding this book right now shows me that you are ready to find another path. You're ready to stop saying no to yourself, your needs, and your boundaries. You're ready to know what you want for yourself and in your relationships. You're ready to create space for peace and ease in your life—enough of that wired-and-tired overfunctioning perfectionist crapola. You're ready to reclaim your true self and remember who you really are.

I'm proud of you for wanting something different for yourself, my perfect little marzipan. Because I believe in the deepest, most essential part of my being that you deserve to know that you are loved for who you are, not what you do. You deserve to feel safe and accepted in your authenticity. You deserve to know your own mind, to trust your own experiences, and to live a life that honors both.

Are you ready to stop putting yourself last, my love?

Let's get started.

Part 1

Foundations of Emotional Outsourcing

Chapter 1

What Is Emotional Outsourcing?

I'll never forget my client Luisa: a bright, successful, charming woman in her late twenties. On paper she had it all together as a first-generation college graduate with a fancy grad degree, an impressive job and great relationship, all the things we are told define us as Successful Women. We had just started working together and one day when she logged in for our weekly call she said, "So, um, Béa . . . I'm so sorry to ask—God, this sounds so stupid—but, um . . . how do I figure out what I want for dinner?"

We both laughed, but I knew what she was really asking: "How do I know what *I* actually want? How do I make decisions for myself? How do I trust that what *I* like matters?" Like so many of my clients, Luisa had inadvertently prioritized the other people and accolades in her life for so long that she lost track of herself, her wants, her feelings—so much so that, unless she had someone telling her what *they* wanted for dinner, she didn't even know what to make.

In the decade plus that I've been supporting women to reclaim their lives, identities, and relationships, I've seen hundreds of Luisas. Vibrant, remarkable superwomen who feel broken—trapped in lives that don't feel like their own, confused about how they got there, and not sure what to do differently. Card-carrying Good Girls who never rock the boat, who are always there to help and never, ever complain. The token woman of color, used to smiling through her colleagues' microaggressions and stifling a scream while she educates her white colleagues yet again, but never letting her frustration bubble to the surface. The overfunctioning oldest daughters (bonus points for oldest immigrant daughters!) who grew up taking on too much, too soon, without support, and never realized that it wasn't their job to take care of the people around them to their own detriment.

Each and every one of these women grew up learning that she was not good enough in subtle or overt ways that she maybe recognized or that lay just below her level of consciousness, impacting nearly every decision without her even realizing it. It's a painful, deep-seated belief that shows up in our lives in ways we're often too busy overfunctioning and people-pleasing to notice. I know, because I've been there, and I'm willing to bet that it's where you are too. If...

- you do for others at the expense of your own mental, physical, financial, and emotional well-being;
- you please everyone except yourself;
- you know what everyone needs and what's best for them...but you draw a blank when it's your turn;
- you're afraid of not doing everything perfectly because, if you don't, they might not love you anymore (or some variation on this story);
- your mood depends on the mood of the people around you;

- you "just know" what someone else is feeling, what they need, and how they're likely to react, but you don't know (or give credence to) your own feelings;
- you've lost touch with your needs, wants, and limits;
- you believe that other people's opinions about your life, your beliefs, your priorities, and the way you live matter more than your own;

...then, my love, you're already familiar with Emotional Outsourcing—my term for the chronic habit of looking to everyone and everything outside ourselves for our sense of safety, self-worth, and emotional well-being, because we do not believe that we are inherently worthy of love and care. It's a painful set of thought habits and nervous system experiences that are all too easy to come by and are the very reason we stay stuck in codependent, people-pleasing, perfectionist patterns that erode our sense of self and only serve to affirm that we are not good enough exactly as we are.

You deserve to live from your authenticity. You deserve a life that feels like it's yours—not a life of painful, self-eroding martyrdom; of chronically attempting to "fix" the people around you; of trying to prove your worth and your value to make people care about you, so that you can finally feel safe. You deserve better than that, *mi querida*. We all do. And I'm going to show you how to get it.

As we take these first steps in our journey to reclaim your sense of self and your conviction that you matter, and to create mutual, nurturing interdependent relationships, we're going to get clear together on what Emotional Outsourcing is, where it comes from (spoiler alert: It's the patriarchy and other systems of oppression along with our family blueprint!), and why its impact on our lives is so darn hard to override.

YOU ARE NOT CODEPENDENT

My darling, let's get this out of the way: You are not codependent and definitely not "a codependent person." Nope. Not a thing. I know, you've probably been told that you are, the same way that you probably get labeled "a perfectionist" or "a people-pleaser," but I want to say loud and clear that these terms are *not your identity*—they certainly don't have to be if you don't want to claim them, and I sure don't. I know this flies in the face of traditional (read: old, unhelpful) narratives, so let me explain.

Historically, codependence has been understood in the context of relationships involving substance addiction (generally alcohol), coming into popularity during the war on drugs in the 1970s and 1980s. I'll use the terms used then here to situate it in that moment: alcoholic and addict (versus the person-first less stigmatizing language I choose now). It describes a pattern in which one partner enables the other's addiction. In these cases, the "codependent" person, often the spouse or family member of an "alcoholic," would become overly involved in the "addict's" life, taking on a caretaker role and attempting to manage or control their behavior. This dynamic allowed the alcoholic to continue their destructive patterns without facing any consequences, since the codependent person prioritized the addict's needs over their own, lying and covering up for them, taking their problems on as their own—ultimately finding a sense of purpose in the role of "enabler."

This pathologizing framework often shifted the blame for addiction-related dysfunction onto the enabling family member—disproportionately wives and mothers—and turned care and empathy into something wrong and excessive. Women were encouraged to blame themselves for their husbands' behaviors and were taught that their emotional investment in others was a sign of illness and disease (which, to say the least, is a vast oversimplification of complex relational dynamics that ignores larger structural and societal factors that contribute to substance use issues, such as poverty, trauma, systemic racism, and the lack of social support services and community supports). Before long, care, empathy, and emotional investment in others came to be seen as wrong and excessive. And by the height of the war on drugs in the seventies and eighties, addiction was framed as a disease in recovery communities, and the psychological patterns of the addict's family members came to be seen as a sort of parallel "addiction" to caretaking and control—a diseased way of relating that needed its own treatment. Yikes! No wonder so many women feel stuck, shamed, and permaeffed. I know I couldn't see myself in those outdated definitions about codependent women being broken, defective "enablers" of their alcoholic husbands. That just wasn't my situation at all, since I didn't have any "alcoholics" in my life that I knew of. I also couldn't accept that codependence was a "disease" to be "cured," and, notably, I wasn't and am not alone in that critique. As it turns out, there is significant disagreement in the psychological literature about what codependency actually is. It's not in *The Diagnostic and Statistical Manual of Mental Disorders*—the current standard for mental health diagnoses—and there is only one psychometric index (a fancy way of describing an evaluation tool) to evaluate whether someone "has" codependency. It's called the Holyoake Index,[1] and the dozen psychologists I have spoken to about it all turned up their noses at it. I would argue that this profound lack of agreed-upon diagnostic criteria exists because codependence isn't diagnosable per se,[2] and that's because it's not a disease, condition, affliction, or psychological issue like depression, ADHD, PTSD, or generalized anxiety.

After a decade plus of research, self-study, study with master teachers, and work with thousands of women on this topic, I do not believe that people are born lacking self-worth, destined to believe that everyone else's feelings, wants, experiences, needs, and general well-being matter more than their own. Unlike the old paradigm, I do not believe that anyone is inherently codependent, and I do not believe that adopting that label as an identity serves us in any way.

When we think of ourselves as "a codependent person," rather than a person who acts from codependent patterns, we deny ourselves the chance to see that we don't have to be this way forever. But when we recognize that codependent living is a set of learned behaviors, rather than a disease or an immutable fact of your personality (ditto for perfectionism and people-pleasing), we open ourselves to the possibility that we can shift and change. If codependent, people-pleasing, perfectionist habits are just that—habits—then we can unlearn and rewire those patterns, the same way we can any habit.

Moreover, it's become clear to me that codependent, perfectionist, and people-pleasing tendencies are, in a way, the same thing, and so it behooves us to see them as such, to heal them together. Getting to the shared root of these super-duper common patterns, "Emotional Outsourcing" is the term I coined (and trademarked going back to January 2012) to describe the way we chronically source our sense of worth, value, significance, and emotional wellness from everyone and everything outside ourselves (to our own detriment), because we do not believe that we are inherently worthy of love and care exactly as we are. It's a super-common set of thoughts and nervous system experiences that leave us tap-dancing for our lovability, desperate to prove that we are good enough, worthy of the care and belonging that all humans need to survive.

Those of us who identify with words like "codependent," "perfectionist," and "people-pleaser" have lost our connection to the three things that every human needs: safety, worthiness, and belonging. Unable to source them internally (i.e., know for ourselves, regardless of what anyone else says, that we are safe with and significant to the people we love and to ourselves), our brilliant minds and bodies work overtime to source them elsewhere. In this way, we *outsource* our emotional well-being to others.

Since it doesn't feel safe or smart to be ourselves, our minds and bodies learn how to become who others want us to be, and over time we learn to live our lives for other people, instead of ourselves. When you're stuck in Emotional Outsourcing, you live life constantly grasping for others to tell you you're good enough. Pretty enough. Smart enough. Accomplished enough. *Enough* enough... and you always come up short. My clients struggle with resentment, exhaustion, and burnout. They ruminate constantly, paralyzed by indecision. They go along to get along. They go above and beyond to please everyone else, thinking it will mean they can be happy too... only to realize that it never really works that way. They fall into relationships because the other person likes them, or stay in lopsided romantic partnerships, convinced they can "fix" their partner, going along to get along, resigned to what is, even when they want something wildly different, avoiding conflict at all costs, and stuffing down all that hurt and disappointment with a simple "I'm fine."

WHAT DOES EMOTIONAL OUTSOURCING LOOK LIKE IN PRACTICE?

Emotional Outsourcing is comfortable discomfort that we learned as a survival skill, often in childhood. It gives us a framework for relating that we believe will keep us safe and connected... at the cost of hiding away our truest, most authentic and beautiful self. When we focus our attention outward, we can't worry about our own needs, desires, and capacity—both because we're spending all our time and energy focused on others and because, well, what if they conflict with someone else's? What if they're inconvenient? What if they make us a burden? Instead, we mask our true feelings and thoughts, abandoning our sense of self until we lose track of our own inner voices entirely. Rather than knowing our own value, we use praise, affirmation, validation, busyness, jobs, responsibility, certifications, marriages, kids, to prove that we are worthy. It's as though we're performing our lives onstage before an invisible jury, doing everything we can to earn their applause and approval.

It's no surprise, then, that we doubt our own voice. By the time my clients find me, they often sound like Luisa—so disconnected from their internal compass that they don't feel like they know who they are anymore. Emotional Outsourcing and self-doubt go hand in hand, and to say we don't believe in or trust ourselves barely scratches the surface. We think, rethink, and overthink every choice, then doomscroll and numb ourselves out just to get a break from the relentless anxiety and shame.

Desperate to feel in control of our lives, we overfunction and overachieve until there's nothing left except resentment toward the people we care about. We learned that our okayness depends on everyone else's, driving us to pour endless emotional labor—especially into our romantic partners and immediate family—convinced that if someone is sad, anxious, or upset in any way, it's our job to fix it. We can't tolerate our loved ones' discomfort, pain, unhappiness, anxiety, any more than we can tolerate those feelings ourselves. Unable to manage our own feelings, and scared we don't deserve to feel better anyway because we're maybe inherently not worthy of love, we do the next best thing and step in to manage theirs.

True to our people-pleasing ways, we chronically take on too much responsibility, which leaves us perpetually overwhelmed—especially since we have to execute each and every one of those responsibilities perfectly, obviously. We blur the lines between our concerns and the concerns of others and lose sight of where we end and they begin. This over-involvement in other people's lives often leads us to neglect our own needs and boundaries and, you guessed it, builds more overwhelm, emotional distress, and resentment, strengthening that core story that we're not safe, don't belong, and aren't worthy of love or care.

This pervasive feeling that we're trapped in a life that isn't ours is suffocating. We don't even realize that we're out to win an Olympic medal in worrying and martyrdom (gold, obviously), and we corrode our physical health, mental well-being, and relationships in the process.

Physical Consequences of Emotional Outsourcing

As a family nurse practitioner specializing in evidence-based holistic medicine, I would be remiss not to mention the myriad serious chronic conditions that we can connect to Emotional Outsourcing. You see, when we prioritize everyone and everything else around us, life feels like a delicate tightrope walk or walking on eggshells, trying to keep everyone happy, which is both mentally and physically draining. Our nervous systems struggle to keep up with the relentless cycle of stress and vigilance, stretched to the limit by too many moons of living with all that adrenaline and cortisol (both stress hormones) flooding our bodies in unbalanced ways.

From lived experience as both a patient and a provider, I know that the chronic stress of Emotional Outsourcing can impact nearly every system in our bodies. The concurrent nervous system dysregulation can contribute to gut issues ranging from bloating to irritable bowel syndrome and small intestinal bacterial overgrowth,[3] disrupt thyroid function (cue fatigue, weight changes, and mood disturbances!),[4] and can increase the risk of heart disease, stroke, type 2 diabetes, chronic inflammation, and so much more.[5]

The stress of Emotional Outsourcing can also disrupt sleep patterns, as much for logistical reasons (you, my perfectionist nugget, are likely burning the midnight oil at every turn to get it all done and are thus not getting enough or consistent sleep) as for emotional ones: Raise your hand if you've kept yourself up at night replaying that awkward thing you said or worrying someone was mad at you. And don't forget the impacts of unbalanced hormones.

All that can make it difficult to fall asleep or maintain deep, restorative sleep, leading to insomnia or fragmented sleep patterns.[6] The stress of hypervigilance, especially when we're not sleeping well, can promote inflammation and a cascade of immune dysfunction, which in turn make the body more susceptible to infections, exacerbate autoimmune diseases, and lead to chronic pain from chronic tension patterns.[7]

All this is to say, the consequences of Emotional Outsourcing are no joke. If you're noticing significant changes to your mood or gut, or you're struggling with your mental or physical health, I would strongly encourage you to make an appointment with a licensed primary medical care provider who can help you start to care for your perfect body, while you do the emotional work we're doing together here.

Folks who develop Emotional Outsourcing become adept at reading other people's feelings—so much so that they supersede our own. We read people's moods like the weather, watchful for the slightest shifts in posture or tone, poised to dive in and fix it. Good Girls and peacekeepers to the bone, we learned that our role was to manage the feelings of the people around us. It's a familiar story: Mom's upset at your sibling and you do something silly to break the tension. Your dad seems stressed, so you pull out that A+ you got on your test, hoping that showing him how amazing you are will cheer him up and take the worrisome (and potentially dangerous) feelings away. As a kiddo, I used to do odd chores around the house like ironing or scrubbing the kitchen floor (which, to be clear, exactly zero people asked or expected me to do), because I could tell that my new-immigrant parents were stressed, and I believed that if I could just create a little more order, a little more peace, maybe the chaos and tension in the house would settle down. Maybe they'd finally relax. Maybe, just maybe, I could feel safe. It was my way of trying to control the uncontrollable, to manage the emotional weather of the house by being the "good kid"—the one who fixed things, even if that meant doing things no one asked for, because in my mind, their peace equaled my safety.

Folks with Emotional Outsourcing habits are professional other-people prioritizers. We notice others, tending to every need, catering to every desire, secretly praying that maybe they'll do the same for us... someday... if we earn it hard enough. I once had a client who told me that when she was growing up, her mother told her that the best relationships were ones where you focused completely on the other person's needs: "You take care of them 100 percent, and hopefully they take care of you too. If they're happy, you're happy, you know?" Scared of asserting our needs directly—which could lead to judgment or abandonment—we muffle our needs under layers of hints, suggestions, and unspoken hopes. And, my love, that's a one-way ticket on the Disappointment Express to Resentmentville, USA.

Underfunctioners can be emotional outsourcers too, but instead of taking on too much, they avoid responsibility, expecting others to carry the emotional and practical load. My ex-spouse was the textbook example—refusing to lift a finger around the house, leaving every bit of emotional labor, planning, and caretaking squarely on my shoulders. It wasn't just about chores; it was the way they simply checked out, outsourcing their emotional needs and life responsibilities to me, as though I existed solely to handle everything they couldn't be bothered with (the way their mother did). It was their subtle way of keeping themselves safe from discomfort, conflict, or growth, while I overfunctioned to keep the entire system running, never realizing how much I was facilitating their detachment and avoiding my own needs in the process.

HOW DID WE GET THIS WAY?

It is so very easy to blame all our Emotional Outsourcing habits on our families of origin. But it's not the whole story, my love. Emotional Outsourcing is born from an attempt to navigate complex emotional landscapes, generally when we're way too small to be doing such things, and is modeled for us by our caregivers and community.[8] The need to live from codependent, perfectionist, people-pleasing stories is one that has been shaped by generations of cultural conditioning in response to systems that thrive on keeping you disconnected from your inherent worth.

The individual factors of how we were parented, our personal history, and our lived experiences absolutely impact how we think, feel, and behave as adults (which is why we're going to spend all of chapter 2 exploring the role of your caregivers). *And!* So much of the reason that Emotional Outsourcing exists in the first place is that this sh*t is in the proverbial water, thanks to three overlapping systems of oppression: patriarchy, white-settler colonialism, and capitalism.

Patriarchy isn't just a system that disproportionately values men and masculinity over women and femininity—it sets the stage for Emotional Outsourcing by devaluing care, empathy, and collaboration, teaching people to outsource their emotional labor in exchange for validation from those in power. Under patriarchy, Emotional Outsourcing thrives because women, in particular, are socialized to prioritize others' needs over their own, to seek external approval, and to tie their self-worth to how well they care for others. Women are told to keep the peace in their relationships, maintain harmony, and shoulder the emotional burdens of others, even when it leads to burnout and resentment. For example, if you feel pressure to be the emotional caretaker for everyone in your life, prioritizing their needs while ignoring your own, that's patriarchy in action. If you believe that expressing your needs makes you "needy" or "selfish," so you push them down and focus on serving others instead, that's another manifestation of patriarchy.

At the same time, it's also the patriarchy that tells men not to have feelings, especially "feminine" ones like tenderness and sadness (anything but rage, really). This dynamic keeps both men and women trapped in narrow emotional roles, with men outsourcing their vulnerability ('cause boys don't cry, remember?) and women internalizing the idea that their worth lies in taking on others' emotional weight.

White-settler colonialism is, at its core, a system of dominance over indigeneity and, by extension, over the land, its resources, and its people. Like patriarchal masculinity, colonialism privileges whiteness in a social and cultural context that colonialism itself created, where those who do not fit the dominant group are judged, controlled, and exploited—and it hurts *all* people, including, yes, white people. Its focus on extraction and accumulation seeps into the smallest details of life, teaching people to view relationships, work, and even their self-worth as transactional and conditional, and fosters a world where millions of people go hungry every night while billionaires exist, all on the same planet that institutionalized colonialist greed is quickly killing. White-settler colonialism builds Emotional Outsourcing into its very foundations, because it conditions people to believe that caregiving, emotional presence, and nurturing are valuable only when they serve the dominant structure's goals. White supremacy leads us to view self-care as indulgent rather than necessary and to see relationships as investments for future favors, not ways to build more loving community and mutual aid; dismisses joy as unproductive or frivolous; and treats the Earth as a resource to be used and abused rather than a living organism to be loved and respected. In short, if you feel like your worth is measured by how much you can offer to others and what they do for you in return, that's colonialism quietly shaping your sense of self and your relationships. It brings a whole lot of tit-for-tat into our lives when loving could just be what we do and who we are, not something we keep score around.

Last but not least, **capitalism** is an economic system based on a logic of accumulation; however, its impact has ballooned far beyond the financial sphere. These days, internalized capitalism has come to shape how we value ourselves and others. Our social capital comes from the accumulation of praise, validation, and success (through competition, not cooperation). As a result, we've come to prioritize doing over being, and we've come to believe that we have to earn and win love, care, respect, and even rest. Treating burnout as a badge of honor? Capitalism. Turning self-care into a commodified industry? Capitalism. Seeing time spent with loved ones as unproductive? Capitalism. Struggling to ask for help from friends because it feels like a burden? Capitalism.

All systems of oppression challenge the three things that all human mammals need to survive: safety, worth, and connection. Together, capitalism, white-settler colonialism, and the patriarchy insist that our personhood is not guaranteed unless we are wealthy, white, and male. You are not of value unless you're producing. You're only worthwhile because you're pleasing to others. You're only as good as what you give. Your sovereignty and self-determination are negotiable, and your status is less-than because you're a woman; fat; queer; Black, Indigenous, and/or a Person of Color (BIPOC); disabled; chronically ill; neurodiverse—anything that "deviates" from the white Western capitalist norms.

These systems of oppression are harmful in their own right and have impacts on our psyches, lives, and relationships that merit books of their own (and many have been written). What I want you to see, though, my love, is that your Emotional Outsourcing habits exist and persist precisely because they are logical, natural adaptations to living under these systems. For example, when you are living in a marginalized body in a white patriarchal society, living as your authentic self is often dangerous, both emotionally and in the most literal, physical sense. BIPOC folks, fat folks, and folks with visible disabilities receive constant and prolific messages about being unattractive, not good enough or smart enough, and on and on. Those messages are often backed with real, material forms of systemic oppression, poverty, discrimination, and violence.

Code-switching or modifying/shape-shifting your speech, behavior, appearance, or way of being in the world to adapt to different sociocultural norms and to make others more comfortable with you is a useful skill and survival strategy long employed by marginalized communities to attempt to find more acceptance and to be safer in the white world. Same goes for masking (in the case of neurodivergence) or closeting yourself (for 2SLGBTQIA+ folks). They are brilliant strategies for getting ahead, for being more "palatable" (such a gross word and experience) at work, or when interacting with systems of power-over like the police.

Adding insult to injury, these systems of oppression train us to think that we—and not the system—are to blame. Women aren't just *called* codependent like it's some kind of personality flaw—we're shamed for it, dismissed as doormats, ridiculed as wallflowers. We're gaslit out of our own reality, told that needing or relying on others is a personal failure. But here's the thing: Until shockingly recently, our dependence wasn't just cultural—it was *legal*. Codified. Enforced. Not a flaw, but the system working exactly as designed. In the United States, women couldn't have homes or bank accounts in their own names until as recently as the 1970s.* Marital laws treated women more like property than people of equal standing with their husbands. Women were not legally required to be part of medical studies until 1993—meaning that our understanding of our bodies was as a "deviation" from men's bodies. As of this writing, women in the United States do not have nationally guaranteed rights to decide their own reproductive healthcare. My love, the very structure of the world that we live in requires us to depend on men and the institutions they've created. What could our mothers, their mothers before

* Dear one, when was your mother born? I promise 1970 was not as long ago as you may think.

them, and their mothers before them do but learn not to rock the boat—and teach you to do the same.

ENDING EMOTIONAL OUTSOURCING IS A FEMINIST ISSUE

We have so much more opportunity today than those women who came before us—and we owe a debt to our feminist foremothers. And yet, and yet, I hear from women day in and day out who feel trapped in their lives, unable to find that mythical balance between the demands of family life, keeping up households, maintaining social bonds, and working full time while also trying to grow as humans and to heal from their own childhoods. Forget enjoying their lives or taking care of their own needs—who has the time or energy?!

For all the progress we have made, women are still socialized to put other people ahead of themselves in almost every context. For this reason, we can't talk about Emotional Outsourcing without acknowledging that it's an inherently intersectional feminist issue. We juggle it all while thinking and believing what we're taught: that other people's needs, moods, wants, desires, and wellness are more important than our own—and it shows. So often girls are socialized to be good, quiet, docile, diminutive, to control and suppress our anger, appetites, bodies, authenticity, to the point where we forget who we are. We're "Mother's Little Helper," training for the day when, as wives, we will meticulously plan every meal, every outfit, every moment of our family's existence, well accustomed to the weight of unvoiced desires and our needs perpetually penciled in for "later." We doubt ourselves endlessly and struggle to make decisions for ourselves (after making a bazillion decisions for everyone else all day). *Of course* we struggle to own what we want and to live our lives on our own terms.

These expectations are invisible by design and become normalized through our socialization and conditioning and the endless demands of our emotional and physical labor. With love and compassion I'll say: Everything is working against women coming to the realization that we've been trained to externalize our sense of worth, value, and importance in life—writ large. We were raised to "be codependent."

You see, systems of oppression thrive by keeping all of us who are living in marginalized identities separated from our lived experience in our bodies, to see our bodies as object and commodity, something to be managed, controlled, tamed—as a problem or vulnerability to distance ourselves from. The powers that be train us to believe them that there are so many, many ways we're not enough, in order to control us and sell us creams, bleaches, treatments, diets, exercise regimes, and so on that might just cure us of the self-loathing they instilled in us. Too busy riding the roller coaster of not-enoughness and unworthiness, we remain detached from our physical bodies, primed to change who we are and how we appear to the dominant cis white male gaze via capitalist consumption (which, by the way, rarely even works to make us feel good about ourselves).

At the same time, women are taught that we are incomplete on our own and what we want, need, and desire in our own lives has to take a back seat to caring for children, partners, parents, and the feelings of every man we encounter. We continue to be asked to define ourselves in relation to others, to see our value only as doers, martyrs, creators, and nurturers—through our roles as mothers, wives, and daughters—never just *us*. In the patriarchy women are seen as "natural caregivers," as somehow inherently more nurturing and capable of offering care, taught that putting others' needs before our own is what women just "naturally" do (even after studies have debunked that nonsense).

Now, am I saying that it's a bad thing to take care of people? Absolutely not. Not for one second. None of that "every man for himself" white-settler colonialist nonsense here. No human is a rock or an island—we need one another. Each and every single human on this planet needs love, care, nurturing, and community to survive. It's natural and so beautiful to take good care of the people we love—to call or text to check in, to do nice things to see them smile, to want the very best for them and support them in their lives. But taking care of others *above* ourselves as a chronic, unconscious obligation is where Emotional Outsourcing rears its ugly head. Doing for others so that they'll think highly of you or need you or make you feel good about yourself isn't caretaking—that's Emotional Outsourcing. It's manipulative without realizing it, and it hurts everyone involved.

As long as women and girls are taught to disconnect from our desires, minds, and bodies, healing Emotional Outsourcing will continue to be a radical, political act. And so long as BIPOC, disabled, queer, femme, neurodivergent, fat, and other marginalized folks think the problem is *us* and not the system, you can bet the farm that we'll all stay spinning in Emotional Outsourcing, *because of course we will.*

WHERE WE'RE HEADED INSTEAD: INTERDEPENDENCE

Most folks think that the opposite of codependence is IN-dependence. And there's a certain logic to that: When you no longer orient yourself around others, who else is there to orient your life around except you? The patriarchy and Western colonialism certainly glorify that rugged individual mind-set, unabashedly making a moral argument that all people can and should pull themselves up by their proverbial bootstraps. But Emotional Outsourcing is an inherently relational issue. We didn't gain these survival skills in a vacuum, and we can't heal them in a vacuum either. Instead, my love, my goal for you—and for all people—is *interdependence.*

Interdependence is a relationship dynamic where two autonomous people rely on one another with mutuality. It's a relationship characterized by a balance of reciprocity—give-and-take, where each party both contributes to and benefits from the relationship, without obligation or keeping score. In the context of personal relationships, interdependence often looks like a healthy dynamic where people who care for one another support each other emotionally as well as practically, while at the same time maintaining a sense of their own identity, capacity, and worth. In other words, you can count on your people to show up for you, and they can count on you to show up for them—but never at the expense of either's well-being.

This is why the work of ending Emotional Outsourcing is so radical: It asks us to take care of ourselves, precisely so that we can be in community with others, while also participating in mutual aid and caring for community as self. When Audre Lorde wrote about self-care in the epilogue of her essay collection *A Burst of Light*, it was never about self-centered independence. As she says, "Caring for myself is not self-indulgence, it is self-preservation and that is an act of political warfare."[9] The endless parade of face masks, bubble baths, and calls for "me time" has stripped Lorde's words of their original meaning. Self-care was always intended to be radical, political, and paradigm shifting. You must learn to care for yourself in order to care for others. And by letting others care for you, you remember that you are lovable. You must rebuild a relationship with yourself to be in true relationship with others—and through healthy connections with others, you learn how you want to relate to yourself. Because in the end, it *has* to be in service of collective liberation—otherwise, it's just the same old oppression, repackaged with better skin and a fresh coat of gloss.

YOU ARE WHO YOU WERE TAUGHT TO BE

My sweetest sweet pea, I say again: Your Emotional Outsourcing habits formed and are challenging to rewire because they came from a super-duper smart place. When you live in a society and a culture that jeopardizes your very dignity; when your safety (psychological, financial, social, physical, mental) is not assured; when your value depends on how much you do or how well you play the roles you've been assigned without your consent (like Good Girl, Perfect Daughter, Selfless Wife, Model Employee, Tireless Caregiver); when you can't count on your community to show up for you unless you're indispensable and constantly "adding value"—my love, no wonder you learned to be vigilant about everyone and everything around you, and to use their needs, feelings, and opinions as the rubric by which you grade yourself. It just makes sense.

Your Emotional Outsourcing habits are not dumb, bad, or evidence of failure—they once served you. Deeply. Pinky promise. But, well, you wouldn't be reading this book if you didn't already see the ways that they were keeping you stuck. Living from our Emotional Outsourcing is like trying to squeeze into an old baby sweater: There's nothing at all wrong with the sweater, or with you, my tenderoni—you've simply outgrown it. It's time to knit a new sweater, and a new identity to wear inside it.

The good news—yes! there's good news!—is that since codependent, perfectionist, and people-pleasing habits are learned and not at all inherent to you, they are also changeable. You do not have to stay in that overwhelm and burnout and resentment forever, my softest bunny. You get to remind yourself over and over that it's not you, it's the system—and find new, powerful ways to show up for yourself and the communities you love. Because no matter how much the world wants us to believe otherwise, I know deep in my soul that your worth does not depend on anyone but you. It's time that you reclaimed that knowledge for yourself. Once we ditch the story that we're broken, we stop fighting for our lovability and hustling for our worth, and start to believe that we're inherently lovable. From that grounded place, we can take real personal responsibility—knowing we're inherently good—which lets us acknowledge when we've done an oopsie (or really effed things up) without questioning our sense of Self.

In part 1, we're going to explore the specific scripts that we learned from our caregivers, how they got written into our nervous systems, and the way shame drives us to abandon our own needs, feelings, and experiences. This is complex stuff, lovebug. Give yourself time and space to metabolize it, and remember—to borrow once more from Audre Lorde: "Nothing I accept about myself can be used against me to diminish me."[10]

JOURNAL PROMPTS
WHAT'S MY BASELINE?

Before we can begin the work of healing Emotional Outsourcing, we need to take stock of the ways in which it is currently affecting your life. Using the following journal prompts as a guide, I invite you to explore how knee-jerk habits like putting everyone else first, overriding your needs, desires, and emotions, or overfunctioning contribute to your feelings of stuckness and resentment in your present life.

1. What do I think of when I hear the term "Emotional Outsourcing"? Does it feel familiar to me? How or how not?

2. How do I feel about the idea that my worth (i.e., how I feel about myself) could come from within, rather than from what others think of me?

3. When have I felt like I needed someone else's approval to feel okay about myself? What was that like?

4. How do I typically respond when someone asks me to do something I don't really want to do or have the energy or capacity to do? How and when do I (and don't I) check in on my capacity?

....

....

....

5. What messages have I received about being "perfect" or "helpful" in my relationships? How do those affect me?

....

....

....

6. In what ways have I been taught that it's important to put others' needs ahead of my own?

....

....

....

7. What do I think it means to "live for myself" instead of living for others? Have I ever experienced that?

....

....

....

8. How do systems like the patriarchy, colonialism, and capitalism impact my day-to-day life? How do they impact the ways I think about myself and my worth?

9. What might be possible if I truly believed that I am inherently worthy of love and care?

10. What feels impossible for me right now? What do I think might change in my life if I started to trust my own opinions and feelings more?

Chapter 2

The Origin of Your Self-Story

We all carry a story about who we are, a self-narrative that shapes how we show up in the world. Maybe you believe you're the smart one, the funny one, the good friend, the "mom" of the group, or the one who can't resist turning a casual outing into a competition.

My client Claire used to call herself "the responsible one"—always the first to volunteer, to solve every crisis, even when it left her depleted. Then there's Maya, who proudly wore the badge of "the peacekeeper." It was her unspoken job to smooth over family tensions, even when it meant swallowing her own frustrations. These stories we carry about ourselves aren't just anecdotes we tell; they're the identities we live from.

Whether it highlights our strengths or amplifies our insecurities, our self-story shapes how we engage with the world around us.

While we are always becoming new versions of ourselves, modifying our stories, growing, and "selfing" (to borrow a term from Gestalt psychology), it is also true that you carry a self-story that was created and shaped in relation to your primary caregivers. The way we were parented becomes our worldview and shapes the stories we carry about who we are; who it's okay for us to be; what friendship, kinship, family, and partnership mean; and what we can expect from those categories of people in the future.

Shifting our self-story is vital to unwinding our Emotional Outsourcing habits, and we need to understand the template we've been living from to make those changes. So, in this chapter, we're going to take a closer look at how we came to doubt our safety, worth, and belonging; understand the role of attunement in creating the self we come to inhabit; and explore how different parenting styles give unique shape and nuance to the story that your inner kiddos have been carrying for you all these years.

A Note about Caregivers

Caregivers are anyone and everyone who had a consistent hand in raising you. Your primary caregivers may have been your biological parents but could equally have been a grandparent, an aunt, a foster or adoptive parent, or a family friend. As you read this chapter, I want you to keep in mind all the folks who spent a significant amount of time as your guardian or caregiver. The way they related to you and, in turn, the way you learned to relate to them will have had a hand in the stories you grew up to tell about yourself.

ATTUNEMENT: THE BEDROCK OF CONNECTION

As children our options are limited. We're pretty acutely aware that we're small animals. Not such great drivers. Unclear on where to get a credit card or how to use money. We're also not so good with reading, and also where does food come from? In short, we know that we are deeply dependent on our caregivers for our survival and that no matter how much we'd like to, we can't leave… so we do what we must: We adapt, we read the room, we figure out how to get our needs met in whatever environment we find ourselves in. We fine-tune ourselves to what keeps us safest—because staying in our caregivers' good graces isn't just a preference; it's a matter of survival.

And what makes a kid feel safe? It's not just about having food on the table or a roof overhead, though those are critical. True safety runs deeper. It's in the predictability of care, the stability of the environment, and the reassurance that their needs—both physical and emotional—will be met. Kids need to know that their feelings are welcome, that they won't be punished or dismissed for expressing them. They need to feel seen, heard, and understood, not just tolerated. They need clear, reliable limits and boundaries and healthy social interactions.[1]

Above and beyond any one of those things, though, is something called *attunement*. Attunement is a caregiver's ability to deeply understand and respond to a child's emotional signals,[2] and it's super-duper important to our tiny, tender, still-growing nervous systems, which need attunement in order to know that we are safe (and likely to stay safe) with our caregivers.[3] One of the earliest and most influential definitions of attunement comes from Daniel Stern, a prominent developmental psychologist. In his 1985 book *The Interpersonal World of the Infant*, Stern described attunement as the process by which parents match their emotional state to that of their infant, helping the child to develop emotional regulation and interpersonal understanding. Picture a parent adjusting their response based on a child's subtle cues, a mom soothing her crying baby, or a dad acknowledging his teen's frustration about curfew instead of just laying down the law. It's the way my client Naomi comforted her grandson after a fall on the playground: Seeing his hesitation, she knelt beside him and in a soft tone said, "It's okay to feel scared after a fall, bud. What if we try climbing together this time?" Her attuned response acknowledged his fear, offering both emotional support and a sense of safety, encouraging resilience and trust in her presence without making it about her and how scared *she* was. It's all about being in tune with another's feelings, creating trust and understanding. Consistent, appropriate, and supportive attunement plays a significant role in shaping and regulating a child's developing nervous system (and is important for trust between adults too!).

I can't overstate this, my love: Attunement matters *so*, so much. Attuned interactions nurture the emotional connection between child and caregiver, building a bond of trust and understanding that lets the nervous system rest in social safety. That in turn boosts the *social engagement system*, a term from Dr. Stephen Porges's polyvagal theory,[4] which refers to the set of neural structures and pathways involved in social connection, communication, and feelings of safety during social interactions. Through attunement, this system is refined, helping children gauge when they're safe to be their authentic selves and when it's time to mask or code-switch. For example, validation and understanding attunement sounds like "I see that you're feeling frustrated. It's okay to feel that way." Curiosity in attunement sounds like "What was the best part of your day today?" or "I wonder why you would say something so hurtful to me—what's going on in your heart?" Consistent loving feedback from attuned caregivers assists children in honing vital skills, including active listening and collaborative play, while having an attuned caregiver as an emotional anchor helps kids better navigate stress, planting the seeds of resilience that flourish over time.[5]

My nerds, trust in one's environment and caregivers is essential for effective stress regulation throughout our lifetime. Brain development is significantly influenced by experience, and repeated attuned interactions can strengthen neural pathways associated with emotional regulation. Over time, a child who consistently experiences attunement will develop a more robust neural network dedicated to recognizing and managing stress and to feeling safer amid life's proverbial slings and arrows. Furthermore, through consistent attunement, we learn that our environment is predictably safe and that we can rely on others, namely, our grown-ups, to rescue us when life gets lifey and scary for our small selves.[6]

When our early environment doesn't meet our emotional, psychological, or physical safety needs, then we are likely to develop coping and survival strategies that are often a setup for the codependent, perfectionist, and people-pleasing habits that we see in Emotional Outsourcing. Take my client Grace, for example. As a kid, when Grace sat politely and silently at the dinner table, she was allowed to stay. But if she talked too much and interrupted the adults, or squirmed in her seat, or made silly faces instead of chewing with her mouth closed (as six-year-olds are wont to do), she got sent to her room without dinner. It didn't take sweet Grace very long to realize that, if she wanted to eat, she'd need to hold in all that excitement and playfulness. Over time, Grace's self-story started to sound like this: "I'm only loved when I'm quiet and well behaved. I can only get my needs met if I don't make a fuss or bother anyone." And that didn't just stay in childhood—it followed her into adulthood, where holding in her joy became entangled with survival. Her nervous system had linked feeling expansive, bright, and fully herself with risking safety, connection, and worth.

ATTUNEMENT LEADS TO ATTACHMENT

You may have come across the concept of attachment styles—a way of categorizing connections between infants and toddlers and their caregivers originally formulated by British psychologist John Bowlby[7] during the mid-twentieth century that has been expanded on (and some parts problematized) by a half dozen researchers since. Broadly speaking, when we receive adequate attunement from our caregivers, we develop a secure attachment. You feel safest when your primary caregiver is near because they are trustworthy, reliable, and a consistent safe place to anchor (which sounds pretty dreamy to me), and you feel safe when they leave because you know they're coming back—they've not given you reason to doubt them. The rest of us, however—and especially those who grapple with Emotional Outsourcing—likely did not receive consistent safe and secure attunement from our primary caregivers and instead formed one of three insecure attachment styles: anxious, avoidant, or disorganized attachment.[8]

Before we get too much further, I want to clarify something my clients are often wildly confused about. "Attachment relationships" are survival-based relationships, namely, those between children and caregivers. Adult relationships, my chickadees, are *not* that kind of relationship. While we do develop relational habits and tendencies that we project onto our adult relationships, I want to invite you to use your attachment habits as a way to understand parts of yourself but resist taking a broad brush to say, "I *am* this kind of attached." Your attachment style is not who you are; it's a part of you. Just like we talk about codependent, perfectionist, and people-pleasing *habits*, I would urge you not to get too cozy thinking of any particular attachment style as an identity. Brains are blessedly plastic or malleable, and we can change our go-to attachment styles when we do the work to overcome Emotional Outsourcing and to reclaim our somatic or bodily connection with ourselves.[9]

Now, kids who develop **anxious attachment** become—you guessed it!—*anxious* about the availability of their caregiver, often fearing abandonment. That fear of abandonment may spill over into other areas of their life, and they become preoccupied with relationships, constantly seeking reassurance and validation, fearing that, without it, they'll be alone, which, to our human pack-animal nervous system, is tantamount to a death sentence.

Avoidant attachment typically manifests in children as rugged self-reliance. Their profound independence grows because their caregivers are emotionally unavailable, unreliable, immature, or neglectful enough that they learn not to trust them or lean on them. They learned early on that showing vulnerability and relying on others can lead to disappointment, so they cut themselves off somatically and emotionally and may struggle to open up to others or to rely on them.

Disorganized attachment is born from a complex pattern of traumatic experiences or an extreme of inconsistent caregiving. Children with this attachment pattern display an unpredictable mix of behaviors that seem contradictory or hard to interpret, a story that licensed clinical and forensic neuropsychologist Dr. Judy Ho, PhD, describes as "I hate you, don't leave me."[10]

One of the many ways people with insecure attachment styles deal with our deeply rooted fears and anxieties in relationships is through Emotional Outsourcing. If you've grown up anxious about the stability of your relationships, you likely become overly attuned to the emotions and needs of others, often at the expense of your own. Folks with an avoidant attachment might also suppress or hide away their needs, emotions, and authenticity, feeling it's the only way to prevent rejection or disappointment, because it certainly was in childhood.

In a relational sense, without a secure attachment foundation, understanding where you end and another person begins can be challenging. You might find it hard to say no, or you might feel responsible for another person's happiness or well-being. Many of us also tend to fear conflict because we understand that there is a superhighway between conflict and abandonment, so we eat our feelings and swallow our pride instead of speaking up when we are hurt or upset.

KIDS BELIEVE THEY ARE THE PROBLEM, NO MATTER WHAT

Recognizing that your caregivers can't, won't, or aren't able to attune to you and that they aren't safe to attach to is an existentially frightening thing for a child.[11] Remember, my darling, as kiddos, if we aren't being attuned to or the parenting we are getting isn't working, we often don't have the option of finding it somewhere else. Children understand the danger in blaming or being mad at our parents, and in the sad alchemy of brains and nervous systems hardwired to keep us safe, we decide that we (a being within our control) rather than our caregivers are at fault when our needs for safety, worth, or belonging are threatened. Those self-stories can sound like anything from "I must have deserved it" or "I just need to ace this and then my mom will be proud of me" to "If I pretend to like this movie, maybe Dad will let me snuggle with him on the couch," and so on.

When young Sheila tried to show her artwork to her busy parents, they barely glanced her way, mumbling a distracted "that's nice" without looking up. Rather than thinking, as an adult might, that her parents were just busy and she could try again later, Sheila thought that her art must not be good enough, that she wasn't interesting enough to her parents, and she'd just have to try harder if she wanted their attention (which of course she did—she was a kid, and all kids need their grown-ups' attention; it's part of the gig). Unconsciously, Sheila came to believe that *she*, and not her parents, was the problem in that situation. And while it's unlikely that a single brush-off in a sea of mindful care will catapult a kid into the land of Emotional Outsourcing, a consistent lack of attunement is a pretty reliable way to craft a *New York Times* bestselling self-story that your realest self is not worth attention. And what's a brain to do but double down and push you to seek validation through over-performing, fixing others, and becoming indispensable and impossible to overlook?! Survival skills, baby.

THE FALSE SELF

Given the shame, self-blame, and pain that come with a lack of attunement and insecure attachment, most of us learn early how to mask or negate our genuine emotions, needs, or identity in order to feel okay, safer, and (fingers crossed!) less likely to be abandoned by the adults in charge of us. But do that often enough and for long enough and you develop a false self: the self we present to the world as a way to keep our true self (who we often don't think we like from a knee-jerk, I'm-not-good-enough place) safer, hidden at the back of the proverbial cave.

While I wish I could take the credit, the concept of the false self originates from psychoanalytic theory, particularly from the works of D. W. Winnicott,[12] a British pediatrician and psychoanalyst, and I posit that it's very much a part of the Emotional Outsourcing experience.

For Winnicott, the false self is what arises in environments where our authentic experiences are consistently overlooked, denied, negated, or devalued. To adapt, kids begin to present a version of themselves that is in line with what they perceive to be the caregivers' expectations. They want a quiet kid? Coming right up! A smart one? A+ only from me! A thin one? I shan't eat again! Over time, this adaptive facade becomes habitual, and we don't even realize we're living our lives as someone else.

Chronic Misattunement Can Be Traumatic

Trauma isn't always a boom-bam accident, war, or a single act of violence or violation, and it isn't just what happened, it can be what didn't happen that should have. Trauma can be developmental—the result of living with parents or siblings who are emotionally immature, physically unwell, or abusive or who have mental health disorders or other struggles. Living in a marginalized body under systems of oppression hell-bent on making you feel worthless can be traumatic. Growing up in homes where there is substance overuse or abuse can be traumatic, including well-to-do homes where the expensive single malt flows. Even parents who "did their best" often caused their kiddos trauma, and that's no diss to them—it happens, no matter how much you loved your little baby bears.

What is so important for you to understand is that trauma—be it developmental trauma, trauma between children and caregivers who should have been trustable, or trauma that shocks you to the core—effs with every single part of who we are and can be. It messes with our identity, authenticity, and sense of self, our capacity to be with ourselves and the world around us in healthy ways, and we deserve to be gentle and kind with ourselves as we slowly, gently heal and grow.

Chronic emotional misattunement in childhood is described as an "invisible ACE" (adverse childhood experience or cause of trauma, here developmental)[13] that can have significant and even devastating effects on our emotional and physical wellness later in life. Many of us with chronic or developmental trauma didn't learn that we matter or that we could feel safe; we didn't have parenting that met us, that valued us as us, that told us that we are okay and good and enough *as ourselves*—so we grew into false selves, leaving our real, true, and authentic selves behind.

I can go on and on about what trauma is, but the take-home is this: Trauma isn't what happened; it's how your nervous system reacted to it. If your nervous system chronically went into overdrive or shut down, if you regularly panicked or disassociated, it's okay to call it trauma. As always, I don't recommend that you make any one thing your identity or let it define your future. Rather, I invite you to use your history of childhood traumas as a driver to get the help you deserve.

PARENTING STYLES AND SELF-TALK

What we've talked about so far happens while we are still forming our very first relationship templates, but we don't stop being influenced by our caregivers when we're in elementary school. The seeds of our self-story are strengthened and refined over the years in new relationships and experiences. Moreover, we don't grow out of those core needs of safety, worth, and belonging—they're the bedrock of humanity, and how we source them only gets more complicated with time. After a while and as we get older, we've internalized them so thoroughly that it sounds like we're telling them to ourselves, rather than hearing them from our parents, but make no mistake: You did not come up with those thoughts and beliefs on your own, peanut. The specific ways that your caregivers expressed their expectations and interacted with your emotional needs and individuality in turn became how you tell *yourself* you need to be to receive love and attention.

Now, Before You Throw Your Parents under the Bus...

My love, I get it. It can be so very painful to see that the root of so much stuckness and hurt and frustration in your life can be traced back to the people who are supposed to love you most and care for you always. It can be a shock to step out of that habitually self-shaming, self-blaming mind-set and notice that your caregivers did, indeed, play a role in the painful stories you've been carrying with you your whole life.

May I humbly ask, though, that you give your parents (and their parents and so on) a bit of grace? It's likely they parented in whatever less-than-optimal way they did because they were copying their own parents, who were copying theirs, back to the big bang. Moreover, they, too, grew up in the same oppressive soup of patriarchy, white-settler colonialism, and capitalism that we still contend with today, though likely without the language and support to talk about and understand it all, and fewer resources to make the changes you get to make for yourself now.

Have all your feels about how they parented, my love! It's essential and oh so normal to get angry about the way you see that your caregivers failed you and to call that spade a spade. It's vital to grieve the care, attention, love, and safety you didn't get as a kiddo, and especially to have your big feels about things like abuse or abandonment. Deny none of the hurt and have your sacred anger. All your emotions are welcome here. And when you're ready for a little compassion, remember that they are people too, just peopling along as best they can with what they've got, and, yeah, you deserved more—both can be true, my lustrous flamingo feather, and I'm not saying you need to forgive them, but maybe it could help YOU to see them as fallible humans doing the best they could to manage their own existential anxiety and dread with the limited skills and nervous system capacity they had.

Classic Parenting Styles

Diana Baumrind's parenting styles serve as a gold standard in the literature. She first popularized the concepts of "demands" and "responsiveness" in the 1960s and '70s, identifying three primary styles: authoritative, authoritarian, and permissive.[14] Later, in the 1980s, Eleanor Maccoby and John Martin[15] expanded on Baumrind's work, adding a fourth style—neglectful/uninvolved.*

* Intersectional feminist critique exposes Baumrind's failure to account for how race, class, and gender shape parenting under systemic oppression. Her model, rooted in a Western middle-class lens, pathologizes survival strategies used by marginalized communities while ignoring the impact of patriarchy and structural inequality, especially

In Baumrind's model, "demands" refer to the expectations parents set for their children, expressed as rules, chores, discipline strategies, and stringent expectations around behavior, academics, and extracurriculars. High standards, discipline, responsibility, and achievement are the focus. While children are supported in developing a strong work ethic, responsibility, and discipline, if there is not a balance of care, children can become anxious, self-doubting, and perfectionistic. Responsiveness is similar to attunement: It's about how well caregivers recognize and respond to their child's emotional needs and individuality.

Authoritative parenting is characterized by a balanced approach that combines high demands with high responsiveness. Authoritative parents set clear expectations and enforce rules but do so in a way that is both nurturing and supportive. They encourage open communication, offer explanations for rules, and take their children's feelings into account. They are emotionally available and sensitive to their children's needs. They validate feelings, provide warmth and comfort during distress, and encourage their children's individual interests and passions. Children raised with high responsiveness and high demand tend to have higher self-esteem and better emotional regulation and feel secure in their relationships.

Authoritarian parenting is characterized by high demands and low responsiveness.[16] Parents expect strict adherence to their rules without explanation or feedback. Obedience and structure are emphasized, often at the expense of emotional connection. These are the "I'll give you something to cry about" and "Don't make me turn this car around!" parents. Perfectionism is frequently the result of this style, because the child fears the

on women of color. That said, the framework gives us a jumping-off point to understand how we got to where we are in our Emotional Outsourcing, helping us continue to zoom out to see the various factors that created this mind-set, continuing to help us see that we aren't defective or broken—we're resilient and adaptive.

punishment or disapproval that follows from not meeting their adult's high standards.

In **permissive parenting** (low demands and high responsiveness),[17] caregivers are lenient and avoid setting boundaries, which often leaves children feeling insecure and untethered. While their parents might be nurturing or communicative, kids who are permitted to run their own show don't feel the predictability and consistency that helps humans feel safe in the world. They're also typically uncertain about their role in the family. Left with only their parents' emotion as a bellwether that they're okay, children of permissive parents often learn to please others as a proxy for purpose and belonging in relationships. This can sound like "I don't want to say no to the kids because my mother said no all the time," but without clear boundaries or limits, children are left without a framework for understanding their needs in relation to others, and without a model for external support that feels both reliable and constructive. As adults, they may struggle with setting boundaries, feel responsible for managing others' emotions, and seek external validation as a stand-in for self-trust and internal stability. Without a model for reliable support, they can also find it difficult to ask for help or recognize when they need it.

Neglectful or uninvolved parenting is characterized by low demands and low responsiveness,* where parents are emotionally distant and provide little attention or care. In my day this was referred to as "benign neglect." Our parents didn't not-parent us because they were being mean jerks necessarily; they just kinda didn't even think to do things any other way. With that said, of course we have to give the grace to parents who work outside the

* Paging Gen X and many a zillennial/varsity millennial: It's us! Yes, I know I'm overgeneralizing—totally—and if you know us, the children of the boomers, we are largely a wild and feral generation of kids who raised ourselves on the proverbial sandlot of life, sans parental guidance or an eff being given about where we were all day as long as we were home when the streetlights went on. I want my fellow feral ones to know you're not alone—I see you, my Kool-Aid-stained latchkey kids! I see you healing from your lack of parenting!

home (because capitalism) and simply can't give their children the hours of attunement or care they want to because their energy is pulled elsewhere by financial need. Regardless of the reason, children of this style raised themselves. Latchkey kids made their own Pop-Tarts in the morning and let themselves into the empty house after school (and def were dehydrated, what with only drinking water fortnightly, and then only from a rusted hose in the neighbor's backyard). They didn't feel valued, validated, attuned to or seen when they were growing up, so they seek relationships where they can feel valued or needed, often at the expense of their own well-being. Attempting to gain the attention or love they missed out on in childhood, they learn to people-please early as a way to attempt to guarantee positive attention might beam in their direction.

Modern Parenting Styles

These days, what I hear most from my clients about their experience of their caregivers falls into three categories: enmeshed parenting, helicopter parenting, and parentification, all styles marked by role confusion and blurry boundaries.

Enmeshed parents are overly involved in their child's life, to the point where the child's identity and emotions are intertwined with the parent's. For example, my client Rachel's mother, Irene, shared all her problems with her, including her complaints about Rachel's father, treating Rachel more like a friend or confidante than a daughter. Irene would tell anyone in earshot that "my daughter is my best friend!" and she truly believed it. To this day they're inseparable, and Rachel knows every detail about her mother's emotional life. The result of being her mother's de facto therapist and stand-in for a healthy adult friendship was deep role confusion. Rachel feels responsible for her mother's well-being and never says no or sets boundaries with her, worried about upsetting her. In many regards, she is more like her mother's mother than her daughter. She struggles to differentiate her needs from her mother's, which makes sense. Children of enmeshed parents don't learn to differentiate their needs, desires, and emotions from their parents', and it's a hot mess of confused roles.[18] Some parents, fearing rejection or a rupture in their child's love, avoid setting any limits at all—allowing their children to treat them with disrespect or even cruelty rather than risk confrontation. The unspoken fear is often that enforcing boundaries will drive their child away, leaving them feeling unloved or abandoned. Children who grow up without boundaries or consequences for disrespecting their parents often develop an inflated sense of entitlement or a deep discomfort with authority and accountability. They may struggle with emotional regulation, expecting relationships to revolve around their needs without reciprocity, or they may develop underlying insecurity—testing limits in search of structure but never finding it.

Helicopter parents are all up in their kid's business, overly focused on their child's experiences and problems, often stepping in to intervene even when it's not necessary and the child could absolutely handle it themselves. This creates a profound codependence where the kid overly relies on the parents, not trusting they can handle life without someone else's input, and the parents source their worth from having their child *need* them.[19] For example, Ashley's parents, particularly her mother, who has never built her own life and lives vicariously through her children, oversee every aspect of her life. They manage her projects at her adult job, intervene in friendship issues, and even chose her career path (she went to her dad's Ivy League alma mater, which she could never have gotten into if he wasn't a trustee). Even though Ashley is now in her thirties, her parents still pay for her car and her mom drives two hours into Brooklyn to take Ashley's car in to get its oil changed, knowing she would never do it on her own—she never does anything to care for herself, her household, or her partner. Understanding that her parents' love is contingent on her acquiescing to their expectations, she struggles with self-trust and doubts her abilities. She avoids taking risks, fearing mistakes that might disappoint her ever-watchful parents, and can't ever seem to make a decision for herself because, well, she's never been allowed to. She has no capacity to manage her emotions, and flies off the handle if she senses criticism or that she's being asked to do something she doesn't want to do, relying on anger and intimidation to get her way, like she saw modeled at home.

Finally we come to the complex issue of childhood **parentification**. Broadly, parentification refers to a kind of role reversal (like we saw in enmeshed parenting, in which the child was the parent's de facto therapist) in which a child becomes responsible for the caregiving or emotional needs of their parent(s) or sibling(s). The term was first brought to light by Ivan Boszormenyi-Nagy and Geraldine Spark in 1973,[20] highlighting two primary types: Emotional parentification happens when a child becomes the confidant or emotional caretaker of the parent, and instrumental parentification happens when a child takes over household tasks or caregiving roles.[21]

Now, many studies show that it's great for kids to have chores—and I personally agree that having kids participate in and contribute to the household is an important part of raising responsible, interdependent humans with a balanced sense of self and commitment to the collective.[22] *However*, while some level of responsibility fosters growth and resilience, excessive parentification can rob a child of their developmental milestones (and the fun of being a kiddo!). There is pressure to meet adultlike expectations, and their value in the household is dependent on their usefulness, not their being who they are. Parentified kiddos often come to believe that being perfect is the only way to be safe, and they deeply fear failing their family, further strengthening the story that they need to have no needs of their own, must never be a bother or a burden, knowing it would be *really bad* if they added stress or disappointment to their family structure. Often, parentified kids internalize the idea that rules their childhood: Love and attention are conditional upon their performance and aren't their inherent birthright.

They often become overly attuned to the needs and feelings of their caregivers, learning to prioritize others over themselves at the cost of their own needs and desires—quintessential Emotional Outsourcing. The role confusion they experienced in childhood has taught them to believe that their role in life is to be a caretaker (which means not getting taken care of, generally speaking—or not knowing how to accept love and care when it's offered). In adulthood, this can lead to blurred lines in friendship and romantic relationships, as the parentified kid often relates to everyone as someone they have to play mom to—their BFF, coworkers, and dates alike.

Decolonizing Parentification

The definition of parentification can seem pretty cut-and-dried, but much of the parentification literature has roots in Western psychological paradigms. When these frameworks are used as a universal standard, it can result in the misinterpretation or pathologizing of non-Western family dynamics. In many cultures, older children naturally assume roles of responsibility for younger siblings or even parents without it being seen as detrimental, and intergenerational living is normal and beneficial to all. Labeling intergenerational care as problematic "parentification" can be an ethnocentric misjudgment.

Moreover, research on parentification has sometimes failed to fully consider gendered dynamics, where girls might be more frequently pushed into caregiving roles than boys (a reflection not of "family dysfunction" so much as a reflection of broader patriarchal norms). It is also essential to note that in lower socioeconomic households, it is often out of necessity that children take on added responsibilities, not because parents *want* to dump tasks on their kiddos, but because they must. Thus the lens of parentification can, at times, unfairly pathologize families for economic circumstances beyond their control. An intersectional lens emphasizes understanding the structural factors leading to children's assuming adult roles rather than just critiquing the family dynamics and throwing stones at caregivers just trying to get through a challenging situation.

So, how can you suss out if you or a person you love was parentified? It's all about how it feels and the impact on the kid. You might try on questions like the following:

- Does the child feel like they don't have a choice? Do they feel trapped, stressed, and exhausted?
- Does the child seem overwhelmed, anxious, or persistently sad due to their responsibilities?
- Do they still get to be a kid? For example, do they get to daydream and color and play? Or do they mostly clean and do adult work?
- Are teachers, counselors, coaches, or other adults in the child's life expressing concern (and not just the white teachers who don't get the cultural context...)?
- Are they in this role alone or in community with other kids or family members, which might give them a sense of collective care and not over-responsibility? (I personally think this is the most important question here.)

It's crucial to remember that context and impact are everything. What might be seen as problematic in one context might be normative or positive in another and might lead a kid to feel super-awesome about themself and their role in the home. However, consistent signs of distress, negative impacts on the child's overall well-being, and a lack of balance in roles can generally indicate that a kid isn't just helping out, they're problematically parentified, and they might be on their way to living in Emotional

Outsourcing. Whether the source of the problem stems from the familial milieu or is structural (e.g., a result of poverty), the impact can be the same on the kiddos in question.[23]

Finally, I'll share what I'm calling dual-reality parenting or image-conscious parenting, which is a phenomenon I have seen in many of my clients and patients living with Emotional Outsourcing. A child growing up with a parent who is beloved by the world—charming, charismatic, funny, adored in social settings—yet cold, distant, critical, dismissive, or outright cruel at home, is living inside a psychological hall of mirrors.[24] The world reflects back an image of this parent as kind, generous, warm, the kind of person who lights up a room. The child, though, knows a different version—one that is cutting, withholding, disconnected or indifferent to their emotional needs. This creates a fundamental fracture in their understanding of truth, trust, and ultimately, of themselves.[25]

Children rely on their caregivers to provide a stable, coherent understanding of reality. But when the person they depend on is two-faced—one way in public, another in private—it sets up an impossible conundrum. The external world reflects back to the child that this parent is good, lovable, and kind, while their lived experience is one of rejection, shame, or invisibility. This creates an early and profound cognitive dissonance—the distress that comes when two conflicting truths exist at once and cannot be reconciled. And because children are wired for attachment above all else, their developing psyche has to resolve this dissonance in a way that preserves their connection to their parent. The only way to do this is to turn the blame inward.[26]

- If everyone loves them, then the problem must be me.
- If they can be kind to others, but not to me, then I must be the reason for their coldness.

- If I were different—better, quieter, less needy, more perfect—maybe I'd get the good version too.

Here, the child's reality splits. The truth they feel in their bones—*this parent is unkind to me, not present with me, unpredictable, or unsafe*—conflicts with the truth reflected by society—*this parent is beloved, celebrated, wonderful.* The child learns that their own experience cannot be trusted. This leads to a fundamental rupture in self-trust and self-perception that shapes their entire way of being in the world.[27]

A child whose reality is routinely gaslit in this way cannot develop a stable, integrated sense of self. Instead, they become hyper-attuned to external cues—watching, scanning, trying to discern what version of their parent they might encounter at any given moment. This hypervigilance becomes a permanent state of being, an embodied sense that the ground is never truly stable beneath them.[28] Having coached hundreds of women who experienced this emotional chasm between home and world, I've seen how folks grow into adulthood unsure of their own perceptions. If their body says *this situation feels off,* but the external world contradicts that feeling, they override their instincts. They second-guess their emotions, dismiss their gut responses, and defer to others for truth. They may develop perfectionist or people-pleasing tendencies as an attempt to control how they are treated. If love and warmth were conditional at home—turned on for an audience but off when the doors closed—they may internalize the belief that they must earn care by being *exceptional.* They may become disconnected from their own emotions altogether, because their feelings were repeatedly invalidated. A child who says, *Dad is mean to me,* only to be met with, *What are you talking about? He's the best!* learns that their own emotions are unreliable, dramatized, or outright false.[29]

Since their internal world has been eroded, children of parents like this often grow into adults who seek external confirmation of their worth. If their reality was never affirmed, they may become deeply dependent on external praise, approval, and validation to feel real or good. They may struggle with deep imposter syndrome, because their childhood taught them that people who *seem* good might not actually *be* good. So they wonder: *Am I actually competent, lovable, worthy? Or am I fooling everyone, just like my parent did?* They may unconsciously replicate the same dynamic in relationships, attracted to people who treat them inconsistently—warm in public, cold in private—because it feels like home. They may become over-performers in work or social life to prove to themselves that they are worthy of love, desperate to be *seen* and *chosen* in a way they never were at home.

~~~

I invite you to take your time with these descriptions and journal to understand how your caregivers' style(s) may have contributed to your perfectionist, people-pleasing, and codependent habits. Above all, be kind to yourself, and, particularly for folks with a trauma history, I recommend doing this work with a trusted professional such as a therapist or a well-trained and certified coach with advanced training in trauma modalities.

I also want you to bear in mind that while these examples paint a clear cause-and-effect relationship, in real life, the outcomes of any parenting style can be influenced by many factors, including a child's innate temperament or constitution, mental health concerns, external influences, or other caregivers or mentors. Caregivers can exhibit one specific style or a combination thereof, and a caregiver's style can change over time, especially as they themself grow and heal.

If you're a caregiver seeing your own style here and cringing, know that healing and growth are possible and that owning your part, taking responsibility, coming correct, and wanting to change are huge first steps in breaking old patterns. You don't have to be perfect, and it's never too late to repair and rebuild your
~~~

relationships with the children in your life. Focus on hearing your kids, apologizing, and changing future actions. Don't make your guilt their problem! Don't get defensive! With love I say: Close your mouth and open your heart so you can really hear your adult children's experience and know that you're doing something right if they're even sharing it.

Healing is a journey, not a destination, and even small shifts in how you show up can create a ripple effect of positive change.

~

My little hummingbird, it's understandable that you've been carrying a story that leads you to chronically seek validation, approval, and recognition from others to affirm your self-worth and decisions, or to make you feel safe and included. In recognizing and understanding the familial origins of these patterns, we can begin to understand and hopefully internalize that we are not to blame for the survival skills that have gotten us to where we are today. You're not broken. You're an amazing and wise human who put two and two together and realized that living from a self-story based in codependent, perfectionist, and people-pleasing habits made the most sense... likely because it actually did.

It's all about sourcing safety—in infancy, childhood, and today, as you find yourself reading this book to help yourself, your family, your clients. The things that we think of as identities, habits, patterns, and ways of being are mostly, at their core, attempts to source safety in the whirlwind.[30]

The ultimate arbiter of our sense of safety, though, isn't just our mind, it's our nervous system. At the same time as your kiddo mind has been forming that self-story, your nervous system has been running in the background, learning what's safe and what's not, creating the mind-body patterns, the neural grooves, that we carry with us into adulthood. Buckle in, nerdlings—that's where we're headed next.

JOURNAL PROMPTS
WHAT IS MY SELF-STORY?

Looking with clear eyes at our caregivers' impact on our self-story can be intense, my love. Take time and space with your journal over the next few days to reflect on the following prompts. The clearer you can be about the origins of your self-story, and what that story sounds like for you, the better you'll be able to begin rewriting it.

1. How did your caregivers (again, not just parents but any and all significant adults) respond to your needs when you were growing up? How did that make you feel about expressing your needs?

   ....

   ....

   ....

2. What kinds of behaviors did you feel were expected of you as a child to receive love or attention? Were there certain things you felt you couldn't do or be?

   ....

   ....

   ....

3. What messages or stories did you internalize about how you needed to be in the world to be safe, to be valued, and to belong? How did this impact your expression of your authenticity as a child? In what ways do you see those stories showing up for you as an adult?

   ....

   ....

   ....

4. Reflect on a time when you felt unseen or misunderstood by a caregiver. How did you react emotionally, and how has that experience shaped your current relationships?

5. In what ways did you feel emotionally supported or attuned to as a child? Are there moments when you realize that attunement was missing? How does this show up in your adult relationships?

6. Take a moment to reflect on how each parenting style described in this chapter might have influenced you. Which caregiving styles most resonate with your experience, and how has that shaped your self-story?

7. How has the concept of "parentification" shown up in your life? Did you feel responsible for your caregivers' emotions or needs when you were growing up? Do you still? How has this shaped your adult relationships?

8. What aspects of your emotional life were wrapped up in your caregivers' needs? How did this affect your ability to express your own needs and desires then and now?

Additional Journal Prompts for Parent Readers

As a parent, you sit with a unique double consciousness: You can see the ways that you were parented as a child, but reading these descriptions can also bring up a lot as you see the ways that you parented or are currently parenting your own children. If this is you, be generous with yourself as you consider these additional questions:

1. What stories do you carry about yourself as a parent? Where do you think these stories originated in your own childhood?

2. How did the way your caregivers responded to your emotions shape the way you respond to your child's emotional needs today?

3. What parts of your self-story or story of your childhood feel like they've shifted since you became a parent? What parts remain the same?

....

....

....

4. What are the unconscious expectations you place on yourself as a parent, and how do these relate to the self-story you formed in childhood?

....

....

....

5. In moments of parenting stress or overwhelm, what stories about yourself as a parent do you default to? Are these stories aligned with your current reality, or do they reflect fears and patterns from your childhood?

....

....

....

Chapter 3

The Trap of Functional Freeze

My patient Julia was a superwoman. Calm and dependable, she did it all and then some—and then some more after that: VP of marketing for a national animal hospital chain, PTA auction chairwoman three years running, and the leader of her daughter's Brownie troop. She was the first person to show up with flowers and a casserole if you were sick or grieving, her whole neighborhood looked forward to her Christmas decorations, and she could get more done in one day than some folks get done in a week. Anytime I'd ask her in clinic how she was doing, she'd say, "Oh! I'm fine!" while it was clear that she was anything but. She regularly maxed out the anxiety medication I was prescribing and shared that behind the scenes she was overwhelmed, couldn't remember the last time she felt *anything* really. She spent hours doomscrolling after everyone else went to bed. She couldn't remember the last time she had a big ol' belly laugh or a really good cry. Her husband joked that she hadn't really attended Family Movie Friday in *years (or maybe ever?!)*

because she was absolutely physically incapable of sitting down for more than two minutes (it was a fact; he had timed her). She was always getting up to refill the popcorn or change out the load of laundry or respond to an email. The situation was untenable, and as her primary care provider, I knew the root of the problem wasn't just in her brain; it was in her nervous system too.

My nerdlings, for the last couple of chapters we've been exploring the ways our family of origin and caretakers, along with our sociopolitical location and identities, set the table for us to develop Emotional Outsourcing as our primary approach to the world. Part of what makes our codependent, people-pleasing, and perfectionist habits feel so deeply rooted inside us is that Emotional Outsourcing is a full-body experience. It's not just the impact of systems of oppression, our family blueprint, or stories and behaviors we learned as children that keep us stuck; the way our nervous systems developed in response to the lack of social and emotional safety we felt as children (even if we didn't consciously understand what was going on) leads us to continue acting from subconscious patterns. Julia's experience is so common for my clients—and I know it was my lived experience for thirty-odd years. When we're living from our Emotional Outsourcing tendencies, we feel revved up enough to go twelve rounds with the Energizer Bunny yet totally divorced from our own needs, feelings, wants, and sense of self. We become frozen to our own emotions and sensations in our bodies, detached from our basic human biological impulses, our internal signals to go to the bathroom, drink water, move our bodies, rest, and so on, and our mental and physical health suffers.

This state, so common in Emotional Outsourcing, is called *functional freeze*, and recognizing its hallmarks (i.e., doing all the things while not being present in the world and especially to our own insides and feels) is vital to your healing, my love. In this chapter, we're going to take it from the top and explore how our beautiful nervous systems work to keep us safe. It's gonna get sciency for a minute. I know that for me (and my clients), learning the science of what's happening in my mind-body helped me to understand that I'm not broken or permaeffed when I check out and go blank or when I freak out before even realizing it and can't seem to figure out why—because it turns out that it's not *me*; it's my nervous system, and remembering that brings me soooo much space for self-compassion.

GETTING TO KNOW YOUR NERVOUS SYSTEM

Your nervous system is an intricate web of nerves, organs, and brain structures whose primary function is to keep you safe in a world that it perceives to be anything but. Connecting your brain, body, and environment, your nervous system interprets information about what's going on inside and around us to assess whether we're okay or whether it needs to sound the alarm. Our nervous system develops its proverbial operating system in early childhood,[1] which means that by the time we're in elementary school, we've already laid down core beliefs around who and what are dangerous, where danger lurks, and how to find safety.

Herein, when I'm talking about the nervous system, I'm talking about the autonomic nervous system (ANS). Often called the "automatic" nervous system, the ANS functions right below our conscious awareness and manages our internal environment—all the things we don't want to have to control manually, like heart rate, breathing, liver and reproductive function, and so on. The parasympathetic branch of our ANS is in charge of conserving energy and keeping us chill (you might have learned about this as the "rest and digest" state back in ninth-grade biology). The enteric system controls digestion, and the sympathetic branch mobilizes us when there's a perceived threat, preparing us to take whatever action will save our lives. If your nervous system is the body's surveillance system, your amygdala is the alarm bell. This almond-shaped cluster of nuclei in the limbic system is constantly scanning for potential threats—long before you consciously register them. It's like an overcaffeinated security guard, making snap judgments about whether something is safe or dangerous. And, let's just say, it tends to err on the side of caution.

When your amygdala senses a potential threat—whether it's a lion on the savannah or your boss raising an eyebrow at your email—it sends a distress signal to the hypothalamus, which then activates your autonomic nervous system, which prepares to book it when we hear a roar on the proverbial savannah or, if we can't outrun 'em, to punch a lion in the nose.

Now, if you're thinking, *Hey, that sounds like fight or flight,* you're right! (Look at you go, smarty-pants!) "Fight" and "flight" are the ways our sympathetic nervous system prompts us to act in the face of danger, and since the turn of the century, psychologists have continued to expand our understanding to include "freeze" and "fawn" responses, equally important players in the nervous system survival drama. "Freeze," a primitive survival mechanism in response to overwhelming or inescapable threat, is, in colloquial parlance, when you play possum. It's a mixed state where you're revved up but also stuck—mentally or physically—playing dead, as it were, in the hope that the T. rex might not notice you and will move along.[2] "Fawn"[3] is a common default in tense situations where our other innate biological reactions to push, scream, or run aren't going to address the threat at hand.[4] For example, if you get called into your boss's office, it probably won't help your chances of promotion to hide out in the bathroom, refusing to talk to her, or scream in response to feedback. Conditioned by societal norms, we clamp down on our true feelings, override the desire to get the eff outta there, and, instead, make sure that the scary thing likes us enough that maybe it decides to keep us around after all, like Bambi batting those eyelashes. When you fawn, your nervous system automatically chooses appeasement over authenticity, because that is what your nervous system has discerned will keep you safe—super smart in its way, especially if you're a femme person living in the patriarchy.

Revving up or shutting down our nervous systems is energetically expensive—it uses a lot of the body's resources—so back in the evolutionary day, fight-flight-freeze was reserved for actual lion-attack-level moments, hostile marauders, environmental dangers, or other immediate physical threats. These days, thankfully, we aren't quite so worried about encountering an apex predator when we walk through the supermarket parking lot, but our nervous system is still just as vigilant and has even more to do to keep us safe.

Now, when we talk about safety, we're talking about anything that could cause physical, psychological, or spiritual harm; jeopardize your resources (e.g., job security or housing); challenge your dignity or sense of self; or lead to being ostracized from a group. We're also talking about anything that goes against those big three systems of oppression that we talked about in chapter 1. Under the exigent eye of the patriarchy, white-settler colonialism, and capitalism, just existing can feel and often is legitimately dangerous for many folks. You don't have to look too hard to find examples: driving or sleeping in your own bed while Black; wearing hijab; telling that guy at the bar you're not interested; holding hands with a same-sex partner; using the bathroom that matches your gender identity. There are often real life-or-death consequences for women, BIPOC folks, queer/trans folks, and anyone with a marginalized body or identity. When your identities or choices are in opposition to the oppressive systems that rule your world, you are, indeed, unsafe in those systems. Period. And your nervous system is absolutely right to be on alert.

Some dangers in our lives are obvious, universal, and objective—think: blood, flood, fire. From the vantage of our nervous system, the important thing isn't whether you "are" safe; it's whether you *feel* safe. As many of us know, those can be two wildly different things, and it all depends on how your beautiful body perceives and interprets the information it receives—a process that we call neuroception.

THE ROLE OF NEUROCEPTION

Imagine, for a moment, that you're out for an afternoon walk. You're ambling down the street, taking in the neighbor's flowers, listening to your favorite *Feminist Wellness* podcast episode, enjoying the sunshine on your face. You turn the corner and see a large dog on a leash walking toward you. What do you feel?

There's no right answer here, mittens. Whether you feel excited, neutral, afraid, or something else entirely, your reaction when you "see" the dog in this thought experiment is shaped and guided by what your nervous system has learned from your experience—a process called *neuroception*.

Neuroception is the body's subconscious system for distinguishing safety from danger. Unlike perception, which is a conscious process, neuroception operates outside our awareness, using our senses to scan our environment for cues. For example, we notice whether someone is smiling with their whole face, whether they have their arms crossed, whether they're speaking with full tonal range or flat affect,[5] and we run all this information through the lens of our experience as a way to determine if we should freak out or not. To return to the dog example: Experiences with your own childhood dog may endear you to the doggo coming your way. But if you were attacked by a dog or a caregiver taught you to be wary, you may feel fear. Alternately, maybe your own beloved dog just passed, and the grief stabs so deep that it threatens to knock you over, and you run away from that emotional pain.

Neuroception is why loud voices feel like love and family to some folks and are terrifying to others. Same with teasing or joking, hugs, joy, and sharing space. What is safe in one setting feels safe because it's been coded that way, and then reinforced and adapted throughout our lives.

POLYVAGAL THEORY: BEYOND FIGHT OR FLIGHT

We are constantly engaging in neuroception, where all cues from our environment influence a bidirectional communication system in our body mediated by the vagus nerve. This system works in concert with other neural pathways to regulate mood and arousal—broadly defined as our physiological and psychological states of alertness, wakefulness, and attentiveness. Known anatomically as the tenth cranial nerve, the vagus nerve wanders* through your body from your brain to your lower abdomen. Thus, the vagus nerve is the physical structure that connects our minds and bodies, governing some organs as well as our mood, energy, and emotional capacity (i.e., whether we're anxious or chill, checked out or checked in).

Developed by Stephen Porges, PhD, polyvagal theory offers a way to describe how neuroception and the vagus nerve drive the way we relate to ourselves and the world, often without our conscious input.[6] While several aspects of polyvagal theory are still debated among researchers, and I have some beef with it myself, I have also found it to be a very useful framework for myself and my clients, and I share it as a metaphor, a tool for us to understand ourselves and others better, leading to ever more compassion, despite the theory's shortcomings.

Porges theorized that as our nervous system registers the world around us as either safe or dangerous, it can automatically move us between three primary states like turning the volume knob on a radio, and, yes, I will be oversimplifying some complex science here:

---

* "Vagus" means "wanderer" in Latin.

1. **Ventral vagal** is the "safe and social" state—we feel connected to ourselves and those around us, present in our minds and bodies, chill and checked in. Ventral means "front" and refers to the front body; it manages facial expression, vocal tone, heart rate, digestion, social engagement, and calm states. We are less likely to engage in our Emotional Outsourcing habits when we're deeply seated in ventral vagal. I mean . . . you can't be present to yourself *and* be sourcing your worth externally at the same time, right?
2. **Sympathetic activation** is a hyperarousal of the nervous system and maps to our familiar fight-or-flight responses. You'll know you're in sympathetic because you feel revved up. Your heart rate and blood pressure go up; your breathing is shallow; your muscles are taut and tense. Your thoughts narrow to the threat in front of you, and bodily functions like digestion and complex thinking pause while your body marshals its energy to protect you—prioritizing only immediate-survival tasks. I teach my clients to be attentive to the "sympathetic thoughts" that alert you to your state: I have to! I have to go *now*! To call him! To figure it out! Now, now, now.
3. **Dorsal vagal** is hypoarousal of the nervous system, the nervous system state of last resort that your body goes to when it's pretty sure you're about to be snacked on by a hungry-hungry hippo. It describes a disconnected, sometimes dissociated, deer-in-headlights state. The dorsal system gets activated when your nervous system says, "Whoa, now, this is *way* too much. I can't physically get away, but no way am I sticking around mentally and emotionally for this." In a dorsal vagal state, you may experience a sense of disconnection or emotional numbing as your body attempts to conserve energy and protect itself from overwhelming stress, like when a lion is coming to

have you for lunch. This can involve changes in pain perception and consciousness as the body's metabolic processes slow down, leading to decreased blood pressure, decreased heart rate, and a numbing or dissociative experience as you become less present to your current experience.[7] When we're shut down or disconnected in dorsal, we're likely to think things like *I don't know* or *I can't* and perpetuate our Emotional Outsourcing with thoughts like *I know this relationship is hurting but I just can't figure my way out*... or *I want to change these habits but it just feels so overwhelming in an exhausting way.*

CLIMBING THE POLYVAGAL LADDER

Deb Dana, LCSW, a leading expert in polyvagal theory, introduced the visual metaphor of a ladder to help us understand how we move through different nervous system states. This ladder concept illustrates that our nervous system responses exist on a spectrum rather than as simple on/off switches. The ladder visual shows that (1) there are gradual transitions between states, represented by the spaces between rungs, (2) we can be in intermediate positions, not just at distinct levels, and (3) our nervous system can move up or down this ladder in response to perceived safety or threat.[8]

Dana's model helps us understand that our physiological responses are more nuanced and fluid than just being in one state or another. It provides a framework for recognizing subtle shifts in our nervous system and offers a way to visualize our journey toward regulation and safety.

In this visual, the ventral vagal state is at the top: This is our most connected state, where we feel in touch with ourselves and the world. A fistful of rungs down is sympathetic: We're feeling unsafe, and our bodies are activating in the face of perceived danger. The lower third is dorsal, on a spectrum from chill and relaxing to collapsed—shut down in our bodies and shut off from our emotions, doomscrolling social media on our phone with the TV on, absorbing none of it.

Let's look at a quick (and somewhat oversimplified) example: Imagine toddler you is chilling in ventral vagal, hanging out all copacetic in the sandbox in your backyard. Out of nowhere, a motor starts up, backfiring, and it is *so loud*! It startles you, and you cry out—eager to source safety and reassurance from a grown-up. But sadly, in this example, nobody comes. Your mom put in headphones to mow the front lawn, and she can't hear you (the lawnmower was, in fact, what startled you in the first place). That lack of attunement, which sadly is par for your course in this example childhood, only ratchets up your fear, and your nervous system starts revving up into sympathetic, preparing you to do whatever little-toddler you can manage to save your life. Fighting doesn't seem so smart (you're pretty little . . . not a lot of oomph in those punches), so you start to run but trip and fall trying to climb out of the sandbox. You're now fully freaked out. Your body is flooded with adrenaline, and cortisol is on the way. Screaming and crying, you try your best to keep running, but your little body is worn out. The terror is overwhelming. Nobody has come to save you, and it feels like nobody's going to—again. You're stuck. So your body starts to prepare for the worst. That knee you bruised? Can't feel it. Where's Mom? Don't know, but something must be wrong *with you* if she didn't come to save you . . . *right?*

Now, in an ideal scenario, your mom came around the corner a few moments later or your other parent heard you crying and ran outside, saw your distress, scooped you up, and showed you love and care. Their attuned, loving attention affirmed that you were safe and released the fear and tension in your nervous system. Perceiving you to be safe now, your nervous system can move out of that dysregulation and back toward ventral vagal.

Humans are meant to shift up and down the ladder, in and out of regulation, guided by what our bodies neurocept or pick up as cues of safe/unsafe from the environment. Meanwhile, to move through life, we often have a wee bit of sympathetic activation without being in full-blown fight or flight. In fact, a little sympathetic activation is a vital thing if we are to get up in the morning, put on pants, and get to doing the day. Ventral vagal with a smidge of dorsal allows us to deeply rest, meditate, and heal, while the other end of dorsal takes us out of presence completely.[9] Full-on sympathetic is panic, maxed-out dorsal is being catatonic, and there is a *wide* range of experience in the middle, within each nervous system state. We're talking about spectrums, not on/off switches in our nervous system. No nervous system state is bad, we need them all, and we are meant to move flexibly among them all. The challenges come when we spend way too much time at an extreme of experience without coming back to our ventral vagal baseline, where we're able to metabolize food and thoughts, and can live our most present lives.

The way we move up and down the ladder is through a process of regulation and dysregulation. We're regulated when we're in balance, able to shift states with grace and ease. Our logical brain and surveillance system (ANS) are communicating and collaborating in harmony. We run, punch, or freak out when it's called for, we chill out when possible and socially connect when the vibes are right, without pushing or forcing anything. We can respond to stressors appropriately, recover from stress quickly, and maintain physical equilibrium. We're dysregulated when that balance is off. We feel our emotions more intensely; we can't think or problem solve as efficiently; communication becomes more difficult; we feel "stuck" in a nervous system state.[10]

In relational terms, being regulated looks like being able to feel the big feels but not let them take over in a way you're gonna regret—like feeling *so* friggin' angry with your partner while still being able to say, calmly, "Babe, I'm really frustrated right now. Can you tell me more about your thought process here?" Or you might be present and aware enough to know you need to walk away, 'cause the anger you're feeling is SO big and you don't want to hurt anyone with it. If, in the same situation, you're buzzing inside, fuming, seeing red, texting them "What the eff? CALL ME!" and yelling the second you get them on the phone, or if, alternately, you just go totally blank, your limbs feel heavy, you avoid their call and then, over dinner, default to, "It's fine. Yeah, I'm fine," while feeling *so* shut down, then, my precious love, you have crossed into dysregulation.

I want to emphasize that regulation is *not* a conscious process. As the cues from other people, our own body, and our environment roll in, our nervous system automatically shifts us between states to help us cope and to ensure our survival.[11] That does *not* mean that what we think can't or doesn't impact our nervous system state because it very much does; however, when something feels too threatening, your nervous system doesn't wait around for you to make a pro-con list before trying to save your life—it shoves you down that ladder because (from its perspective at least) your life really does depend on it.[12]

Dysregulation Isn't Inherently Bad

My delightful, perfectionist-minded courgette, PLEASE TAKE NOTE! Being dysregulated is not inherently bad. Again, moving between regulation and dysregulation is part of being human. Being Zen and chill and never stepping even one toe outside ventral vagal is *not* the goal of living a human life or healing your nervous system. You're not messing up if you're not in ventral vagal all the time—I just can't say that one enough!

Spritzes of adrenaline and cortisol from sympathetic activation enhance physical and cognitive performance, lend vitality and excitement to enjoyable activities, and give you the physiological boost you need in a real-life dangerous situation (good luck trying to cross a street in New York City or Buenos Aires without it!). On the flip side, there is no deep rest, no end-of-yoga-class Savasana, no meditation, no daydreaming, without dorsal rest—ditto choosing to tune out your uncle's political views at the Thanksgiving table.

Being able to regulate is about being able to choicefully and compassionately call yourself home to ventral vagal when you want or need to. It is not, I repeat, *not* about controlling which states you are "allowed" to be in. Authenticity is the name of this game—remember, my sweet one? My goal for you is to build a loving, trusting connection with yourself and your body that allows you to hold space for dysregulation and all its discomfort, and to build the skills that allow you to shift the state you're in on purpose.

THE WINDOW OF CAPACITY

One of the most important things I work on with my clients is understanding and honoring our capacity. Those of us who struggle with Emotional Outsourcing learned to live beyond our limits from such a young age that many of us don't even recognize that we're doing it. We've become so focused outward that we don't even recognize our own nervous system states and experiences, let alone when we've stepped beyond our limits and into dysregulation.

Celebrated clinical psychiatrist Dan Siegel introduced the term "window of tolerance" to describe an optimal zone of arousal or nervous system activation where we can function effectively, remain grounded, and fully engage with life without becoming overwhelmed or flooded in our nervous system.[13] In my own work, I prefer to use the term "window of capacity," which we'll use here, or my absolute favorite, "window of bodily dignity," which captures something even deeper—our ability to exist in a state of self-respect, presence, and agency without collapsing under stress or overextending ourselves to our own detriment. This framing shifts the conversation from mere survival—what we can *tolerate*—to what actually honors our body, our needs, and our well-being. So often, those of us with Emotional Outsourcing habits have developed an extraordinary tolerance for discomfort, over-giving, and even mistreatment, but that doesn't mean it serves us. The *window of bodily dignity* helps us recognize the difference between enduring and thriving, between white-knuckling our way through an interaction and remaining fully present in our body with a sense of choice and self-respect. For myself and my clients, it has been game-changing to shift the focus from "How much can I take?" to "What can my nervous system *hold* in this moment without becoming dysregulated?" This centers our capacity—our ability to stay regulated and resourced—rather than measuring success by how much we can withstand. It's about caring for ourselves rather than pushing our limits to the breaking point.

Regardless of the terminology, this window in our nervous system represents what we can cope with and still remain in ventral vagal. Translation? This is our comfort zone. When you're in your window of capacity, life feels pretty okay and you can roll with the punches—the epitome of Buddhism's "supple bamboo bending in the wind" metaphor. When something is too frightening, too much, too unsafe, our nervous system catapults us out of our window and into dysregulation so that we can stay safe.

The size of our window of capacity naturally fluctuates throughout each day depending on the ebbs and flows of what's going on in our lives and in our bodies. For example, it tends to be wider, meaning we have more ability to stay present when life gets lifey, when we've had adequate sleep, nutritious food, physical activity, and positive social connections and we've engaged in self-care practices such as mindfulness, meditation, prayer, or journaling. Conversely, it may narrow when we're stressed, sleep-deprived, or experiencing physical or emotional challenges. Trite as it sounds, being hangry can be a pretty handy *ejemplo* for us: Food is an essential survival need, and when our blood sugar dwindles, we get more easily frustrated by way less input. A little extra traffic on the way to drop off your youngest at dance class? Most of the time, no biggie. But at 4:45 p.m. after sitting through meetings so nonstop that you barely had time to inhale a handful of M&M'S? Oh boy . . . your ability to cope with BS is so very narrow, and everybody had better watch out!

Same goes for conflict with your partner. Maybe you're having a calm, connected conversation after a good night's sleep, and you're in your window—able to listen, reflect, and respond, not taking it personally, globalizing, or catastrophizing—wins all around. Now imagine the same situation after a stressful day, no food, and zero time for yourself. Suddenly, their words feel like an attack, and you snap back defensively, making the smallest thing mean everything bad ever, all at once. Your window has narrowed, making it harder to handle the situation with grace. Wild, right? And sooo useful to know when we're working toward more loving, interdependent living.

It's also important to recognize that systems of oppression—racism, sexism, ableism—are stressors that can shrink our window, often without us even noticing. If you're constantly navigating a world that feels unsafe or unwelcoming, your window may be tighter than the window of someone who isn't facing those external pressures. It's not just personal, it's systemic, and knowing that is part of learning how to care for your nervous system in a world that can be brutal.

So, how do we keep that window open and flexible? It's all about nervous system care. Tools like deep, slow breathing, grounding exercises, and self-compassion (all tools we'll be looking at in detail in part 2) help expand the window, along with going where it's warm and spending time with people, animals, plants that are resources for or friends to your nervous system.

Trauma and the Window of Capacity

The vagal brake is a mechanism that allows us to smoothly transition between states of arousal and calm, from freaked to chill. It's most effective and reliable when it has been developed through early childhood experiences of co-regulation, when there are safe people who create ongoing and reliable experiences in the safe and social state of ventral vagal. The Adverse Childhood Experiences Study (ACES) consistently shows that having at least one safe, trusted adult during childhood can significantly buffer against the negative impacts of adverse experiences, even in cases of multiple adverse childhood experiences or other risk factors.[14] That adult can be a crossing guard, bus driver, librarian, or teacher if not a family member or caregiver.

When our nervous system has a well-worn neural groove to ventral vagal and a vagal brake honed in a safe, consistent, loving home, we are able to tolerate distress more easily because we have more cushion from the good (or okay-enough) things in life.

Sadly, trauma can weaken the vagal brake, narrowing our window of tolerance or capacity. What might otherwise be small moments of distress become substantial challenges and state shifts—life getting lifey feels *so* much lifeier for us. Folks with trauma have more of a firefighter's pole than a ladder to those other states, and we tend to stay in those dysregulated survival states longer because we don't have well-worn (neural) paths to get ourselves out of the mire.

If you have a trauma history (be it acute, chronic, or developmental), you're not alone, my love. It is possible to heal and expand your window of capacity—though your journey may require more patience and more self-compassion. In the meantime, please remember that you are *not* broken. Your nervous system is just doing its very best to help you survive, exactly as it has done every day of your life.

FUNCTIONAL FREEZE

Our bodies are amazing. Resilient, adaptive, and wise—we can leave and return to our window of capacity time and again over the course of a day, and the wider that window, the easier life feels. The bummer is that codependent, people-pleasing, and perfectionist habits tend to be associated with having a narrow window, born from a lifetime of hiding ourselves away, of living as a rock and an island (instead of interdependently), from the additive effects of stress or trauma both big and small, and so on, which means we're easily freaked out by small inconveniences or shut down by things like someone looking away while we're telling a story with emotional charge for us. When we chronically live outside our window of capacity, we can end up stuck in something called functional freeze.

Functional freeze is a chronic mixed nervous system state that's part sympathetic and part dorsal, and its rallying cry is "I must but I can't." It's an exhausting tired-but-wired blend of action and inaction, where your nervous system is both activated and immobilized. You're outwardly anxious, busy and "productive" by Western social expectations. That "can't sit down, too much to do!" kinda energy rules your life. Meanwhile you're frozen to your own feels, not connected to your internal experience because you're so outwardly focused. You're doing everything that needs doing (and then some!) but not feeling much of anything... except maybe anxiety, self-doubt, and some wicked neck and jaw pain. You're speaking but not connected to your own words, smiling but not really feeling the joy. It's as though you're thinking your feelings rather than feeling them in your body. Those big, deep feelings? They kinda don't compute. It's as though you're living with thick glass between you and the people around you—watching them be "real humans" while you play the part.

My client Emily used to struggle with this big-time. She often found herself at lunch with friends whom she'd known for years, but as the only single gal in the group (something her mother and, let's be real, the patriarchy were quick to remind her was Not Okay), as soon as the topic of husbands and children came up, something within her shut down. She joked and laughed along at the antics of a toddler who couldn't pronounce their *t*'s screaming "FUCK!" every time she saw a truck on the road, nodded solemnly as a friend complained about her husband's gambling habits, following the social script to the letter... but none of it really reached her heart.

While we look like we have it all together, at our core we're overwhelmed by life and all the feelings that come with it, though we often don't even know we're overwhelmed because we're so numb to it—barely hanging on and living chronically outside our capacity, at a loss for what living in our dignity could even begin to mean. We want nothing more than to lie on the couch and stare at a blank wall for the foreseeable future, to check out and not feel the feels or engage with a life that is just *way, way, way* too much right now. But thanks to what we learned about safety as kiddos, we know it's our job to Look Busy, to be hypervigilant about what people think about us, to make sure we are pleasing people, and to do our utmost to guarantee they find nothing about us that isn't amazing and perfect and oh so lovable... Which definitely rules out couching—so we make it our job to look busy. Thus the "functional" part: We're not catatonic in shutdown or dissociation, so we are, by medical/psychological terms "functional"—yet we're numb enough to our real experience (the part that's too tired, too stressed, too angry, too sad, too burned out, too disappointed by life) to keep going through the motions, frozen to ourselves and life.

This was me to a T: I spent the first thirty-five-ish years of my life in a functional freeze, totally disconnected from my self as a way to survive. I tap-danced for my lovability at every turn, convinced that I had to achieve, perform, and please others to feel okay about myself. I got a medical degree in a subconscious attempt to gain my father's approval, I got married to a person I wasn't attracted to who was cruel to me, abusive in so many ways, because, well, they asked and what was I gonna do, *say no?!* Come on, now. (Furthermore, who am I to mind those 473 red flags waving all around them? I saw them and wrote them off, each and every one.) I was going through the motions of life, rarely if ever actually present in the room I was in, and when I would do things that got me into my body, like go to yoga or dance classes, I would find myself on the floor, sobbing and sobbing, often with no clue why I was crying... other than that I deeply hated my life and the endless patterns I kept repeating, and I had no clue how to change a damn thing. After a lifetime of Emotional Outsourcing and years of cowering from a screaming and gaslighting spouse, I was deeply frozen to my feelings, and so highly exhausted from my A+ gold-star overfunctioning, having married an underfunctioner to boot, as one does. I never sat still, never paused, never stopped. I did everything for everyone, while resenting the hell out of them—and I was even numb to that until it came to a massive head. I kept moving forward, doing and doing as though that could help me outrun the dread I felt deep in my bones—the subconscious aching fear that I was unlovable and unworthy, a bother and a burden, things my spouse was more than happy to tell me on repeat.

Unable to be authentic with myself or others, what could I say except the words every emotional outsourcer keeps on speed dial: "I'm fine. I'm fine. I'm fine." And I was so out of touch with my real feelings that I couldn't have told you anything different.

Folks stuck in functional freeze often appear very "high functioning," which again is not a flex. We become the ultimate overachievers, meticulous planners, perpetual caretakers. We're the colleague who's always on their game, the friend who's relentlessly upbeat, the partner who's ever reliable. We're swimming all out against the current of everyone's opinions, needs, desires, and expectations without really knowing why we're swimming or where we're headed, not ever letting ourselves feel how bone-tired we are because, well, if we stopped, we'd drown.

So the pattern continues: We race around doing all the things we learned to do to get love, care, respect, or validation, so disconnected from our inner voice and emotions that we don't (even can't) know what we're feeling in the moment, almost as though we're on emotional tape delay. My client Angelina is a perfect example. Every Friday she'd smile and nod self-deprecatingly through family dinner, only to explode in the car on the way home—railing against all the insensitive things her parents had said, sobbing as she felt the judgment and shame of her mother's sidelong glances and commentary to "take it easy on the garlic bread tonight," the resigned frustration of never quite knowing how to explain once and for all that being an athletic trainer at the local university was a perfectly good career. Whenever we talked about this pattern, she expressed confusion: Why couldn't she just say what she was thinking in the moment? Why did her mind go blank when they started in on her? Why did she not stand up for herself? She felt confused, and I saw a tender nervous system that was doing its very utmost to keep her true self safe.

What Angelina experienced at the dinner table with her parents was the weight of her nervous system's foot on the brake:

the dorsal side of our functional freeze. Dorsal serves us by disconnecting us from being in the here and now. We don't have to think or do or feel the physical, emotional, or spiritual pain thanks to the flood of our body's natural painkillers (endogenous opioids).[15] While the freeze response can have a litany of physiological and emotional consequences (numbness, lethargy, a sense of disconnection from one's body, feelings of helplessness, worthlessness, or being trapped), freezing is a nervous system's easiest way to minimize emotional damage when it's pushed beyond the beyond.

Angelina's body knew that it was way smarter to not have feelings in the moment. Or generally at all when she was with her family. Her parents weren't going to change their point of view or meddling habits, and they weren't really listening anyway. Why would she go through the pain of voicing all that hurt and disappointment and anger when it would just get her told to "get over it"? Better to shut it all down before they could, at least temporarily.

In my experience, if you keep your emotions and the truth of your lived experience shoved down long enough, eventually you stop feeling them. Some of my clients don't even register their fear or anxiety anymore, and many if not most of the women I work with don't register their anger because we've been taught it's not okay for women to be angry. We've been cut off from our emotional experience for so long that we've disconnected from anything other than full-on-plague-of-locusts-level bad...and sometimes we're not even hip to *that* level of red flag—I know I wasn't—I saw them waving in the wind and kept moving forward anyway. The lights are on, all the guest rooms have fresh sheets and toothbrushes galore under the sink in case someone forgot theirs, there's food in the fridge and a meal plan for the week... but *you*, my love, are nowhere to be found. No one is actually home.

Somatic Self-Disconnection

In my work with clients, I've been known to use the terms "functional freeze" and "somatic self-disconnection" interchangeably. The latter sounds fancy, and I coined it as a way to emphasize the way that this mixed nervous system state causes us to quite literally lose touch with our physical selves ("soma" means "body" in Greek). As a holistic family nurse practitioner and primary care provider I saw daily what happens in our bodies when we live with chronic nervous system dysregulation: mood imbalances, fatigue and weight issues, chronic pain (especially in the jaw, hips, and neck), memory issues, headaches, fertility challenges, autoimmune and thyroid issues, weakened immune systems, and *oh* were there gut issues. So many gut issues. Irritable bowel syndrome, small intestinal bacterial overgrowth, heartburn that wouldn't quit, plus the mystery bloating, parasites, and so on—I had it all and I saw it all in my patients.[16]

You see, when the body goes into dysregulation, most of our "non-vital" bodily systems get put on hold. Gastrointestinal, endocrine/hormone, and reproductive systems? Those are not particularly important if you're about to be TigerSnax™; immediate survival functions are all that matter.[17] Your body prioritizes sending energy toward your muscles, which stay tense and at the ready. Even your diaphragm—the muscle that separates the thoracic cavity from the abdominal cavity, aka the breathy bit—braces, leading to short, shallow breaths, becoming a muscle of stability instead of a respiratory muscle.[18] This kind of breathing disrupts the balance of gases in the body and can actually exacerbate feelings of anxiety and panic, creating a stress-inducing feedback loop between the mind and the body.[19]

Beyond nervous system dysregulation, actively suppressing emotions can have its own significant impact on our mental and physical health.[20] When we consistently avoid expressing or processing our feelings, it doesn't make them disappear, no matter how hard we wish it would. Instead, this emotional avoidance can lead to increased psychological distress and may manifest in higher rates of anxiety, depression, and overall reduced psychological well-being,[21] as well as psychosomatic disorders, where psychological distress manifests as physical symptoms[22] such as headaches, digestive issues, muscle tension, and other stress-related ailments. Repressed emotions also lead to difficulties in relationships, decreased life satisfaction, and coping mechanisms that don't actually serve us (aka "mommy juice" while doomscrolling, overeating, overexercising, or whatever gets you through). Emotional suppression can affect memory, decision-making processes, and overall cognitive function,[23] while increased activation of the stress response system can contribute to lot's of different health issues over time.[24]

All this to say, my love, that being out of touch with our internal experience—our emotions as well as the sensations in our bodies—can have real consequences for our physical and mental health. Psychosomatic doesn't mean "fake"; it means that the mind and body are deeply interconnected, and psychological stress, emotions, or unresolved trauma can manifest as real, physical symptoms in the body. It reflects how our nervous system, beliefs, and experiences shape our physiological state—sometimes causing pain, illness, or discomfort, even when there isn't an easily identifiable structural cause. This doesn't mean the symptoms are imagined; they are very real, highlighting the intricate ways our mental and emotional landscape impacts bodily function. Somatic self-disconnection has kept you "safe" for all these years, but nobody (and no body) is able to sustain it forever. In order to heal and to feel truly well, we have to be able to feel our feels, however slowly we need to.

I'm sharing all this science to help you really believe me when I say that you are not broken, *corazón*. Functional freeze is the natural, logical, *expected* outcome of growing up in a family and in a world that told you that you were not enough as you are and that you cannot and should not expect safety. It is not your fault, and besides, your nervous system didn't exactly ask your permission. By design and evolutionary necessity, our nervous system works without our conscious input—and it will keep doing that until you learn how to intervene proactively on your own behalf to bring yourself back home to you.

JOURNAL PROMPTS
MAPPING YOUR NERVOUS SYSTEM

Nervous system mapping is one of the most effective tools I use with clients to help them understand their body's reactions to the world. It's a way of connecting the sometimes invisible dots between the sensations we feel in our bodies and the states of our nervous system. Often, we respond to stimuli we don't even consciously recognize, and by the time we notice, we're already deep in the reaction. By mapping these experiences, we start to recognize the signs before we've lost our cool or have to apologize for snapping at someone when we didn't mean to.

Your goal for now is just to notice. Once you start working with your mind and body (we're coming for you, part 2!), you will be able to exercise more choicefulness and more agency around how you move up and down the polyvagal ladder. Just as importantly, you'll start to widen your window of capacity (meaning that not quite so many things feel scary and, by extension, fewer things will send you into sympathetic activation or dorsal shutdown, or keep you stuck in both).

As always, my tenderoni, I'm going to invite you very strongly to do this without judgment. Curiosity only! Self-recrimination will not serve you in this process. Once again and louder for the folks in the back: You are not broken! Your nervous system is performing exactly as it should. You can't heal hurt with more hurt, so don't be a meanie-pants to you, please.

Now, let's dive in.

I want you to call to mind a number line that stretches from -10 to 10. This spectrum maps the breadth of our nervous system experiences.

Dorsal Vagal	Ventral Vagal	Sympathetic
-10	0	10

At one end of the spectrum is the dorsal vagal state, which represents total shutdown. This is where you might feel frozen, dissociated, numb, where being catatonic maps to –10 on our scale. This is the extreme end of immobilization, where there's no energy to respond or react. It's like your body has gone into full power-save mode. At the other end is the sympathetic state: the zone of activation, where everything is alert, keyed up, and potentially anxious. The farthest point of this state,

+10, is full-blown panic. Think of a moment when your heart is racing, your breath is shallow, and your body feels like it's buzzing with energy that's about to spill over and you are at a loss for logic, calm, or grounding—full-on panic. At the midpoint—0 on our map—we find ventral vagal. This is where we feel grounded, connected, calm, and able to engage with the world. It's the state of social connection, where your nervous system is signaling to you, "We're safe here; we can be open."

Most of us don't live at those extreme edges of the scale and don't even visit; life happens somewhere in between. The real magic of nervous system mapping is that you don't notice just the big signs (e.g., you had a panic attack or you dissociated for a while), but also the subtler cues in your body that tell you you've left ventral vagal, which, remember please, isn't necessarily a problem. Maybe your hands feel slightly colder, or you start to clench your jaw without realizing it. We can plot those physical sensations all along our spectrum to more clearly identify our level of nervous system arousal (i.e., how worked up or shut down we are).

Nervous System Arousal Levels

Dorsal (shut down)

-10 = Complete shutdown. Inability to engage with surroundings, despair, numbness and heaviness in the limbs, cold or clammy skin

-8 to -9 = Moderate shutdown. Low energy, feeling disconnected from others, lack of motivation, dulled physical sensations

-5 to -7 = Mild shutdown. Difficulty concentrating, avoiding social interaction, decreased interest in activities, mild aches or pains, general fatigue

-2 to -4 = Slightly below calm. Low enthusiasm

-1 = Near calm but slightly withdrawn. Mild disconnection or a sense of being "off" or disengaged; energy is still balanced, but there's a slight withdrawal from full engagement; you might feel a tinge of isolation or fatigue creeping in, perhaps a desire to be alone but not from a place of overwhelm; there's still functionality, but with a subtle pull toward retreat or rest

Ventral Vagal (safe and social)

0 = Calm and relaxed. Balanced and present, consistent energy, steady breathing, normal heart rate, sensation of lightness or buoyancy

Sympathetic (fight or flight)

1 = Near calm but slightly activated. Slight increase in energy, vigilance, and muscle tension; mild undercurrent of restlessness; fidgeting or feeling a touch more reactive to environment

2 to 4 = Mild activation. Increased alertness, elevated heart rate, "on edge" but manageable, neck and shoulder tension

5 to 7 = Moderate activation. Noticeable anxiety, difficulty concentrating, feeling overwhelmed, sweating, tension in chest

8 to 9 = High activation. High levels of panic and anxiety, irritability or anger, racing thoughts, shaking, shortness of breath, pounding heart

10 = Extreme activation. Intense panic or terror, chest pain, hyperventilation, dizziness, urge to escape or engage in aggressive behavior, extreme sensitivity to noise or touch

Everyone's physical experiences will vary slightly, and I invite you to get curious about your physical sensations. For example, my client Colleen knows that when she's bailing on plans last minute because she just *can't* and she's feeling foggy, she's well on her way to a -7 dorsal state in her nervous system. When my client Priya notices that she's moved from pen tapping to constantly checking the clock in a meeting, she's shifted from a 1 or 2 to a solid 3–4 of sympathetic activation. The more we practice noticing these small shifts, the more we can create space to support ourselves, stay present, and engage with life in a way that feels more grounded and intentional. In time and with practice, you'll be able to choicefully intervene before your nervous system combusts and create sustainable expansion in your window of capacity. And fear not: In chapter 6 we're going to learn a suite of somatic tools that will help you do just that.

For now, your mission is to make time at least twice each day to check in with yourself and map your nervous system state. You're going to do that by journaling two things: (1) What is happening for me in the moment? and (2) What is my nervous system state right now? This exercise will be especially effective if you reflect on moments that were especially stressful or overwhelming during your day.

For example, Breeshia did her morning check-in just after she'd corralled her kids out the door and onto the school bus. She noticed that while the chaos of the morning was starting to fade, she still felt some remnant of the rushing, super-focused energy and frustration and described her nervous system at a +2.

Before bed, she thought back over her day and remembered the roller coaster of overwhelm and subsequent numbness she felt after a surprise call from her mother that afternoon, which had made her late for an important meeting. She remembered feeling colder than usual in the conference room and had difficulty concentrating on the present, and she'd canceled her lunch so that she could take a quick nap alone in her office. She mapped that experience as a -5 in her nervous system.

Again, my love, there are no bad nervous system states. Change starts with awareness, and getting in tune with your nervous system will put you back in the driver's seat of your experience.

Finally, I want to remind you that leaving ventral vagal can be a perfectly lovely thing. Maybe you're cozied up on a soft couch with a friend and a cup of tea, feeling relaxed and connected—what you might call a gentle -2 toward dorsal, but still well within ventral's orbit. Or maybe you're at a concert, absolutely *stoked* as your favorite band takes the stage—a solid +4 sympathetic, but rooted in ventral. You're not anxious, you're *alive*.

That kind of nuanced mapping is important work, but it's not where we're starting today. Right now, our focus is on what's keeping us dysregulated—so we can begin shifting toward something softer, steadier. The deep, nourishing work of mapping *awesome* feelings? That comes later, my darling chickadee.

Nervous System Arousal/State Tracker

What Did I Feel in My Nervous System When...

Situation

....

Nervous System State

-10 -9 -8 -7 -6 -5 -4 -3 -2 -1 0 1 2 3 4 5 6 7 8 9 10

Situation

....

Nervous System State

-10 -9 -8 -7 -6 -5 -4 -3 -2 -1 0 1 2 3 4 5 6 7 8 9 10

Situation

....

Nervous System State

-10 -9 -8 -7 -6 -5 -4 -3 -2 -1 0 1 2 3 4 5 6 7 8 9 10

Situation

....

Nervous System State

-10 -9 -8 -7 -6 -5 -4 -3 -2 -1 0 1 2 3 4 5 6 7 8 9 10

Situation

....

Nervous System State

-10 -9 -8 -7 -6 -5 -4 -3 -2 -1 0 1 2 3 4 5 6 7 8 9 10

If you'd prefer a printable version of this tracker, you can find one on my website at www.beatrizalbina.com/statetracker.

Chapter 4

Shame and the Self-Abandonment Cycle

Ah, shame. The monster that lives under the bed, in the closet, and in our hearts—oh so pervasive in Emotional Outsourcing. You know by now how both your caregivers and systems of oppression taught you that you, my turtledove, were not okay as you. You also now know how your nervous system responded by dropping you out of ventral vagal, so often into functional freeze, to stay safe. Shame is the engine that leads us to turn our backs on our true selves time and again, a cycle that bleeds over into our habitual relationship roles and patterns and leaves us stuck in relationships that don't serve us (or, frankly, anyone).

My perfect tender ravioli, I want to say first and foremost that there is absolutely nothing in the world wrong with you. Nothing at all. Pinky promise. Please do not shame yourself for having shame, yeah? My goal for you in this chapter is not to pile on, but rather to start seeing where your shame came from, how it leads us to abandon our true needs, wants, feelings, and experiences, and how all that is manifesting in your current relationship patterns.

THE GLUE OF EMOTIONAL OUTSOURCING: SHAME

Shame is a powerful, painful experience stemming from the belief that one is fundamentally flawed or inadequate, especially in the eyes of others, and therefore fundamentally unlovable.

I deeply believe that we are all born perfect, complete and whole, and I decline to believe anything to the contrary. Through painful lies passed down through families and societies, we've been taught to believe the falsehood that we are broken at our core, when in reality, we are inherently brilliant. It's the structures and systems around us that instill a sense of unworthiness, not any inherent flaw within us. Chronic, toxic shame warps our sense of self, telling us that we are undeserving of connection, telling us that we are unacceptable to ourselves and others, and feeding us the belief that our very existence is flawed. Living with chronic shame is the difference between believing you made a mistake and believing you *are* a mistake.

My client Tasha had one of the sharpest inner critics I'd ever encountered. On the partner track at her law firm, incisive, dedicated, and detail oriented almost to a fault, Tasha was respected by her colleagues. But every time she wrote an email, she broke into a sweat. No matter how clear and concise she knew it to be, as soon as she hit send, a familiar cold shock slithered through her chest. *You should've worded that better. You probably missed something important. They'll think you don't know what you're doing. You're not Ivy League. Your dad doesn't golf with the managing partner. You have to be three times as good as everyone else.* She tried to shake it off, but the voice was insistent, twisting in her mind. *You always make little mistakes. Why didn't you triple-check it? Or have someone read it over for you? Someone who* actually *knows what they're doing. You know you have to be four times better than everyone else. They know you don't belong here.* Her pulse quickened as she clicked back to reread the message, scanning every line, convinced there was something—anything—she'd done wrong. *You're never going to be good enough. You never get it right. You're a fraud.* Even when there was nothing she could find to fix, the knot in her stomach refused to loosen.

So many of us have these cruel voices in our minds, *mija*. We live with them day in and day out, so familiar to us that we don't see how vicious they really are. Shame is the voice that tells us that we are unworthy of love and belonging. It whispers that there's something we've done, lived through, or failed to do that makes us unworthy of connection.[1]

Importantly, shame isn't a tool we learn to use all by ourselves. Just like all of our Emotional Outsourcing armor, it's taught to us over time by our caregivers and the world around us. Children have no way to know what is normal or okay unless it is clearly communicated to them ('cause they're new here, remember?), and a lack of clear communication can confuse them about what is safe and unsafe, what is laudable and what will get them in trouble. We do our best to figure it all out by listening closely to the adults around us, so when caregivers struggle with shame in their own lives, from their own family blueprint, religious upbringing, and so on, we often absorb those lessons by osmosis. Take my client Kimberly, for example. While nobody explicitly told her she needed to be a certain size, Kim's judgmental (size zero) mother often commented on the weight of every person around them, saying things like "Does she really need to eat that? I mean... *look at her!*" within earshot of humans in bodies larger than her own. There was no mistaking her mother's disdain for any body that wasn't super slim, and what could Kim do but internalize that perspective? She lived in fear that a passerby might be thinking less of her unless she stayed skinny, and she subconsciously feared losing her mother's love if she didn't keep herself slender.

Shame can be instilled in us at home and/or by systems of oppression, which thrive by keeping us disconnected from the power that comes from being present in our bodies and secure in our identities, honoring the truth of our own lived experience. It makes a lot of sense, right? People living in their dignity recognize when they're being mistreated or taken advantage of; know and are able to honor their innate worth and subsequently speak up, fight back, demand rights, and say *no* loudly and publicly; and thus are way harder to wrangle into submission. In an attempt to maintain their power, these systems keep groups of folks *they* marginalized in a state of self-doubt and submission through generation upon generation of shame. Beliefs are just thoughts you've heard over and over again, and man do they ever make sure we hear about which bodies, skin colors, desires and sexual orientations, gender, abilities, socioeconomic statuses, and so on are "good"* and which are evidence of moral failing, unworthy, deplorable, and never, ever good enough.[2]

Sadly, organized religion and shame also go hand in hand for many of us, in large part because of our reliance on these traditions to set our moral compass. Religion's influence on women's perception of our bodies is deeply entwined with its doctrines of purity, modesty, and self-discipline, often interpreted in ways that stigmatize natural bodily functions. Many friends, clients, and patients raised in a variety of religious backgrounds have told me they never learned about their periods, sex, even how digestion works, other than when being taught to be deeply and profoundly ashamed of having a body—especially a female body (and that "boys will be boys"). Religious emphasis on needlessness, self-sacrifice, obligation, and the fear that just existing could mean you are out of step with the rules only pile shame onto those tiny emotional-outsourcing-prone shoulders until, well, what's a kiddo to believe but that they are inherently broken and bad?

---

* Spoiler alert: rich, straight, white cis male.

No matter where you learned it, or what you learned to be ashamed of, the sick feeling in your stomach, the tension and anxiety in your body that shame engenders, helped make sure that your behavior stayed in line with what your smart mind and body learned would keep you safe, valued, and included—even to your own detriment.

SHAME WAS YOUR SHIELD

I'm going so say something radical and potentially annoying: As much as it was terrible and *is* terrible and sucks so damn much… your shame was an amazing gift. I know, I know—hold on before you start writing the hate mail. Only a handful of years ago the idea of being grateful for something that made me feel like crap about myself and trapped me in an abusive marriage would have gotten a swift "Eff you!" full-New-York-salute, double-birds-flying reaction from me. But, my love, it's true—what happened was terrible, and your shame was a gift because it kept you safe. Does that mean I'm espousing some "your trauma was your greatest teacher!" kind of #PositiveVibesOnly garbage? Absolutely not. I deeply, deeply wish none of us lived through the trauma of shame, as I wish my own body had not been the site of trauma. Trauma was not required for us to grow or to become more resilient—it shouldn't have happened, end of story. And that said, since it did in fact happen, what I'm positing is this: Your body wrapped shame around you like a soft blanket to protect your tender heart when it was the only option it felt it had. That blanket is the gift, my love: that your body did what it could to love you best.

To be clear, I get that the concept of shame as a protective mechanism[3] can seem counterintuitive, especially given how painful and even debilitating shame can be. But even at its worst, shame forms a protective barrier for our bruised hearts, minds, and spirits. It takes us out of presence and away from ourselves, emerging as a painful first line of defense against criticism, rejection, or abandonment—experiences that send your nervous system spiraling down the polyvagal ladder, negatively impacting your sense of safety.

Take my client Lena, for example. Eager to make new friends, she decided to attend a colleague's birthday party and promised herself she'd talk to at least three new people. Halfway through a story about her new watercolor class, Lena felt her stomach drop. *You're rambling,* the voice hissed. *They're just being polite. No one actually thinks this is an interesting story. Watercolor is a dumb hobby, and look at them, they're wearing a leather jacket—why would you think they'd be interested anyway? They're way too cool for you.* It didn't matter that everyone wanted to see pictures of what she'd painted. Her inner critic already had her on the retreat, convinced that she wasn't good enough for the group and withdrawing before they could reject her. It was a pattern she was familiar with. Her family had moved so many times as she was growing up that she'd learned that it was better to be a loner than a loser; better to sit alone than have people tell you there wasn't space at their table.

As we talked about in chapter 2, kids would *way* rather believe that they are the problem than entertain that their caregivers, the people standing between them and the inevitable forthcoming lion attacks, are anything other than perfect (or good enough to save them when needed—fingers crossed!). And so kiddos internalize shame (I'm the problem for: having needs, feels, health problems, etc.) as a way to make sense of their caregivers' shortcomings because believing that they themselves are inherently flawed and at fault can be less psychologically threatening than acknowledging that their caregivers are failing them or are coming up short when it comes to making them feel safe, like they belong or are worthy of unconditional love and care.[4] Makes super-sad sense, right? This internalized shame becomes a core part of our self-identity and starts us on the road to Emotional Outsourcing as adults—desperately seeking safety, belonging, and worthiness wherever we can source it.

In codependent thinking, shame acts as a regulator of behavior, and we learn to hyper-focus on others' needs and desires in an attempt to avoid the painful feelings of doing something or being someone that your people don't like. When we are primarily valued for meeting other people's needs or for not being a bother by not having needs ourselves, when our value as a human (aka our dignity) is contingent on caring for others, we can come to have a deep-seated fear of abandonment or rejection if we "fail" in these roles.

Similarly, in perfectionist thinking we can have an internalized belief that our worth, safety, and belonging are based fully on achievements (tap-dancing for our lovability) or the absence of mistakes—it's called "*perfection*ism" after all, not "*más o menos*–ism,"* right? So when we did something as horrifying as get a 96 percent on an exam, or when we had a big feeling and our parent tells us we "made them sad," or when we express excitement and joy and someone says, "Calm down, you're being too much," we feel shame, and that shame catalyzes the story that you *did* something bad into the belief that *you* are the thing that's bad. Same goes for people-pleasing strategies, where shame motivates us to continuously adapt and respond to others' needs at the expense of our own. The looming fear of disappointing others leads us to live in accordance with others' expectations, with the underlying shame driving this adaptive but ultimately self-neglectful behavior. Think of shame as a kind of really harmful but also protective social glue that keeps us from doing things that might annoy or inconvenience the people around us, which is vital when their opinion about you matters more than yours.

Internalizing shame can also be an essential way for folks to navigate oppressive systems like the patriarchy, colonialism, or capitalism with less friction (on the surface anyway). Adhering to

* *Más o menos* means "more or less" in Spanish. This is a bilingual joke. I hope you find it amusing.

norms and expectations (even when they are harmful or oppressive) can sometimes be a means of protection against more direct forms of harm or marginalization—like actual violence. When you're in a hostile or potentially hostile environment, shame helps you anticipate the worst and ward against it by masking, code-switching, modulating your gender or other presentation, and generally chameleoning to the situation at hand. Painful as it is, hiding away aspects of one's identity that would otherwise be openly criticized or attacked in a given sociocultural context is a form of self-preservation that need not be, well, shamed, but rather, honored for the act of self-love it is.

THE SELF-ABANDONMENT CYCLE

The tragedy and brilliance of shame is that it leads us to disavow our true self—whom our wise mind and nervous system have come to see as a liability—in favor of the versions of ourselves that *will* keep us safe. In other words, we learned to step away from our authenticity in service of our survival. Little you smartly learned, in subtle or overt ways, that being yourself didn't get you the love, attention, care, or community you needed (yes, *needed!*), so you tried on being someone who might be better received. Desperate to feel safe and regain an illusion of control over our circumstances, we start to entertain the myth that "if I can just fix what's wrong with me, I can keep everything else in line." It's a painful thought—especially because, well, there is truth to it. When we shape-shift into the person others want us to be, they do, in fact, tend to like the "new and improved" version better because it aligns with their story about what keeps *them* safe—and you being moldable and controllable, you being who they believe you *should be*, feels safer all around to them.

The more you see that the person you are at your core isn't valued, cared for, or welcome, the more shame starts piling onto the myths we carry. Over my decades of coaching I've noticed that all of us have a handful of painful inner narratives that propel our false self forward. Following are examples of what they often sound like, and of course yours may not be listed exactly or might be a variation on these—read on with an open heart:

- I don't matter. Not the real me at least...all that matters is/are my looks, weight, accomplishments, grades/job, and how I reflect on others—like my partner or parents.
- I'm only valued if I can manage everything and everyone around me. Besides, I don't want to have to clean up the mess that I *know* will come if I let go of control for even a second.
- I can't show weakness or vulnerability; it's a sign of failure. People respect strength, so I must appear strong, no matter what I'm feeling inside. It's also *way* too dangerous, emotionally, to let others see my feels because they'll use them against me—no friggin' way.
- My big feelings aren't safe—they'll upset or hurt others—so I can't be angry or disappointed, frustrated or sad, and sometimes it's not even okay/safe to be too happy (because if they're upset they'll reject or abandon me, they'll stop loving me).
- If I make a mistake, it proves I'm not good enough, like they always said. If I'm perfect, I can avoid criticism and rejection, so I'll just have to be flawless to be accepted and loved.
- If I keep the focus on them, they won't ask questions about me, which is great because I don't really remember who I am and I'm scared that who I am is inherently bad, so I get anxious when things are about me. Better to keep the focus on everyone else—I'm also way less likely to get hurt if they don't really know me, so...better this way for sure.
- I'm fundamentally flawed and unlovable, so I need to work myself to the bone at school, my job, home, the

> gym. Achieving and constantly improving myself is the only way to earn the approval and affection of others, as it won't be given freely.

At every turn, these stories demand that you turn away from your authentic needs and experience and adopt a new way of being or acting. The result of all these shame stories is the logical conclusion that it's okay for us to be anyone except ourselves. Each time we act in ways that bring up shame and self-criticism, we feel bad about ourselves and go into overdrive stuffing down our authentic needs, feelings, desires, and experiences. It's a cycle of unwitting self-abandonment so second nature it feels like breathing.

My client Melanie felt this constantly as a new mother. On a rare (and much-needed) solo trip to the grocery store, she found herself thinking back over the morning with her son, Luke. He'd thrown a tantrum that morning when she wouldn't let him wear his pajamas to day care, but she knew it wasn't really about the pajamas—he didn't want to be separated from her. *What kind of parent are you, leaving him with someone else just so you can—what? Buy Cheerios by yourself?* She gripped the cart tighter, her throat tightening. *Other moms know how to handle this.* She pushed the cart forward, but the voice kept digging, relentless. *You didn't spend enough time with him today. He'll remember that. He'll grow up with attachment issues just like you did and it'll be all your fault.* Mind racing, breath shallow, she couldn't justify leaving him in day care just so she could go to the kickboxing class she'd been desperate for just a few hours ago. She shoved down that grief, that tightness in her heart and her body, and called the day care—she'd be there soon.

When we live from Emotional Outsourcing, each time our own needs—solitude, rest, company, support, nourishment, or water—come into conflict with the (real or imagined) expectations of others, we push ourselves to the side. Even though overriding and abandoning ourselves can breed resentment and pain in our relationships, it still feels safer than risking our sense of safety and significance. We subconsciously privilege the needs, feelings, priorities, and beliefs of other people over the intuition of our true selves. Instead, and without even realizing it, we step into a variety of Acceptable-and-Safe™ personas—false selves we custom build in response to our environment, which I call our Survival Selves.

SURVIVAL SELVES

Survival Selves are the identifiable personas we adopt to go along and get along. There are a million ways we adapt them to suit our personalities, homes, and cultures, but I commonly see five main archetypes among my clients: Saint, Scapegoat, Martyr, Fixer, and Victim. Each one is a manifestation of a common thought error* that became your personality and approach to life. As you consider each persona, remember to be kind to yourself, okay, chickadee? These thoughts may be "errors" in our grown-up lives, but to six-year-old you, a thought like *I have to be absolutely 100 percent perfect 100 percent of the time or my parents won't love me or pay attention to me* may have just been a fact. No shame here, love, just insights.

You may notice you primarily lean into one persona, or perhaps components and skills of a variety of Survival Selves come up in different settings with different people. Regardless, my love, please take note! These Survival Selves are skill sets, not labels or identities. Each one represents a constellation of actions, feelings, behaviors, thoughts, and stories—a habitual way of coping that those of us caught in Emotional Outsourcing tend to step into. But it is *not* who you are—just like you are not a codependent, a perfectionist, or a people-pleaser. We explore these Survival Selves as shorthand, not as diagnoses, and I invite you to explore with the intention of seeing your learned, wise survival skills for what they

* "Thought error" here refers to a belief you learned growing up that just isn't true, doesn't serve you now, or gets in the way of peace, ease, and joy in life.

are: tools you adopted to feel safe in a world that told you that you are not good enough.

The Saint

Whether you grew up with parents who were highly critical and emotionally immature, or only seemed to pay attention to you when you were the best or worst at something, you likely arrived at the same conclusion: To be cared about and for, you needed to become whatever your caregivers called perfect (which might not line up with your own idea of perfection, but that's beside the point). From a young age, Saints live from the thought error that if they do absolutely everything right—never break a rule, always mind their p's and q's, know exactly what to do at all times, conform to any and all societal norms—then and *only* then will they be enough and, thus, safe.

In a culture that frequently equates worth with achievement (because capitalism et al.), we may believe we have to be perfect to be valued, which of course leads us to constantly seek validation and external markers of our success. This can hit doubly hard for women, particularly those from marginalized backgrounds, who may feel the need to be super perfect in order to overcome multiple biases.

Turns out, though, that perfect is no more achievable than touching the horizon, and the desperate, unending quest to be safe from even a whiff of criticism can leave you like my client Serena, the eldest daughter in a financially strapped first-generation immigrant household who struggled with chronic anxiety, a wicked case of heartburn (and a worse case of burnout), gallons of credit card debt from trying to keep up with the proverbial Joneses with the right clothes, nails, and phone that she actually can't afford, who was paralyzed anytime she had to make a decision for herself from her own true desire (not just following others' example, because, well, what if it wasn't the "right" answer?). To say she distrusted herself barely started it, and jeez-oh-Pete did it show up as self-righteous judgment of everyone and everything they did, à la "So, actually, what you should do is . . ."

The Scapegoat

Kids tend to believe that whatever is limiting the love, connection, and appreciation they crave from their caregivers is their fault[5] (because science), but the Scapegoats take it to the next level. Folks living in this Survival Self learned early on to feel responsible for others' faults, fuckups, and feelings and to always bear the brunt of the collective frustrations,[6] regardless of whether they are at fault or were even in the room when what happened, happened. In my home it was the "joke" that everything was my fault—there would be a sound way off in the distance and the whole room would look at me and make some painful comment that left me feeling like a constant effup—I was made the Scapegoat.

Scapegoats take on pain, anger, and culpability that doesn't belong to them in an attempt to defuse or regain control over frightening or tense situations: *If I say it was my fault, they won't hit my sibling . . . It's my fault my partner doesn't have his medication and isn't feeling well. He said he was going to pick it up, but I should have reminded him or maybe just done it myself to be extra sure . . . I told Mom I couldn't have lunch with her today, but now she probably thinks I don't care about her. I should have just rescheduled my day; it's not like I was doing anything all that important. What's wrong with me that I ruin everything?*

The Scapegoat survival style is rooted in internalizing blame, creating an illusion of control—after all, if you're causing the problems, you can fix them, too . . . right? "My fault" becomes a default way to protect against the never-ending dread that maybe you *are* actually a completely garbage human. By making themselves the problem, they attempt to maintain peace, hiding their authentic self to avoid the vulnerability of being seen. This strategy offers a false sense of safety, as they sacrifice authenticity for the illusion of control, staying trapped in a cycle of guilt and self-blame.

The Martyr

The Martyr lionizes self-sacrifice, leaving most of themselves behind—their needs are nothing when everyone else needs so much! It's true that loving generosity is a beautiful thing—but when you give so much so hard for so long (and to everyone and anyone who comes across your path) that your entire identity becomes sacrifice . . . you've crossed over into martyrdom. Martyrs feel safest when they are indispensable—this is the woman who brags about how busy and overworked she is, while taking not-so-secret pride in being "the one who holds everything together."

A child who sees their primary caregiver constantly giving everything for the family, never prioritizing their own needs, might internalize that endless sacrifice is the "right" way to express love and devotion—it's what Good Girls and Good Wives do for sure. Moreover, folks with Martyr Survival Selves have internalized that they only have a place in a given social unit (work, family, romantic partnership, friends) when they have something to offer. Pile on a little societal praise, and it's little wonder that so many folks socialized as women believe that our worth is tied to our sacrifices. Adopting a Martyr Survival Self can lead to relationships where one person constantly gives (aka overfunctions), generally to their detriment, while the other just takes and takes (which is also to that person's detriment, though that's a little harder to see at first blush). Overwhelming resentment and thoughts like *Why am I the only one who does anything around here?* are foundational to Martyr relationships, and they tend to make sure everyone knows they're killing themselves on your behalf.

What folks don't see when looking at this style without the lens of Emotional Outsourcing is that the Martyr Survival Self is about the performance of giving as a cover-up for shame and a loss of connection with embodied dignity. *Ósea*, they *do* and *give* and *sacrifice* at all times, but they're gripped by a subconscious fear that if they stop giving, they'll be seen as dispensable, unworthy, and forgotten. Unlovable. It also bears mention that the pull to the Martyr persona is compounded for BIPOC women and others from marginalized communities, who might feel compelled to sacrifice themselves for the greater good of their community. There's a reason the stereotypes of the Strong Black Woman and the Selfless Madre Latina are alive and well.

The Fixer

The thought error of the Fixer is that *if I know what to do and how to fix it, people will see that I matter enough to be worth saving in a fire, or when the lions come to destroy the village... If I'm useful, maybe they won't reject or abandon me.* Take my client Jo, for example: The youngest of four daughters to an overwhelmed single mother, Jo came to believe that her value lay in being the problem solver, the one with all the answers. She had a deep-seated fear of being seen as irrelevant or unworthy that, in adulthood, subconsciously drove her to overstep boundaries to *insist* on telling the people around her what they needed to do to fix whatever was plaguing them—whether they wanted her input or not!—and skillfully avoided confronting her own issues by always being the advice giver.

Because Fixers' status as saver-of-the-day depends on others being a hot mess, they often find themselves with high-drama friends or partners, in work situations where things are a cluster-cuss, entwined with folks who are sick, in the throes of substance use issues, or otherwise in need of someone to swoop in to save the day. Fixers do an awful lot of swooping in, and they're usually the first ones to abandon their own projects to make you soup and tea at the first whiff of a cold, even when they have a major deadline tomorrow—which, by the way, they'll be sure to let you know they put off to take care of you.

While I find the narrative that casts people with codependent tendencies as inherent "enablers" overly simplistic and dangerously devoid of social context (and has generally been used in quite a misogynistic manner), there's no denying that the Fixer archetype can indeed fall into enabling behaviors. In their quest to be indispensable, a person with Fixer habits may inadvertently perpetuate dependency in those they "aid," discouraging self-sufficiency and personal growth. This is the crux of enabling: It's not a matter of assisting someone too frequently or generously; it's a pattern of interaction that prevents others from facing and dealing with their own challenges and consequences (thus robbing them of the chance to grow and learn).

The Victim

The Victim survival style isn't about actual victimization from external factors, but rather a survival-driven adaptation of a position in a relationship dynamic. That is, it's a conditioned stance that of course comes from having felt helpless at some point in life, typically in childhood, where you learned that to get attunement you had to exaggerate your distress. Through the magic of kid-brain, folks living as Victims believe that they only matter when they are suffering and so *of course* it feels safer to step into the persona of someone who is always in crisis. The squeaky partner, parent, or friend gets the attention, right?

The person in this role generally feels helpless, oppressed, or unable to improve their situation, often despite having the means to do so. They say things like "Ugh, I just can't catch a break!" when confronted with any challenge, or often use statements like "You just don't understand how hard it is for me" in conflicts as a way to subconsciously shirk responsibility.

Susan was impossible to talk to. Her daughter, my client Zoe, tried repeatedly to tell her how she was feeling, to explain that it hurt her when Susan didn't know the names of her friends or ask any questions about her new life in college. But, wrapped in her Victim persona, Susan couldn't hear her. "You have to understand how hard this is for me!" she'd hiss, tears in her eyes. "I just sent my only kid away to school and now I have nobody. If you could just understand where I'm coming from, you'd see that me not remembering everything about your new roommate isn't that big a deal—you wouldn't make this all about you. I'm going through a massive change!" After eighteen years of Susan taking center stage, Zoe finally got the message that her life wasn't as important to Susan as her own suffering, and she stopped even trying, sharing nothing with her mother beyond the absolute necessities, like when her flight was arriving home. Meanwhile Susan, so wrapped up in her own suffering, blamed her daughter's "independent streak" for the lack of intimacy in their relationship and never asked Zoe what was going on. Susan lacked the capacity in her own nervous system to show up to attune to her daughter's, and the relationship suffered greatly for it.

While it can seem like folks in Victim mind-sets are self-absorbed, selfish jerks, intensely and solely focused on their own lives and suffering, it's not that cut-and-dried. They've found an adaptive way to escape what, in their experience, was even greater suffering—suffering they faced when they were more fully themselves. In the fun-house mirror of our brains, the learned helplessness of adopting a Victim persona is preferable to being rejected, ignored, overlooked, and dismissed—all experiences that invalidated their dignity and set off the alarm bells in their nervous system that things were now officially Unsafe. The more a Victim leans into these disempowering, self-sabotaging behaviors, the further they get from their authentic agency and capability, and sadly, the more they push others away, which just strengthens their story of aloneness and suffering.

The Confidence Paradox

Confidence may seem at odds with shame, yet it's a false-self trait that we *love* to rock. Many of us living with codependent thinking are outwardly very confident people, know-it-alls even, and yet we feel fundamentally unworthy and use our confidence as a cover-up to try to get people to see the razzle-dazzle of our charisma, and not the heartbreak of our self-doubt. Confidence gets us validation and approval (which our nervous systems believe equal more safety) so we learn how to appear confident, how to be very attractive, charming, interesting, curious, smart and well-rounded, funny, and charismatic people and just try to keep that whole low-self-worth thing behind those curtains.

Think of confidence like putting on your best party mask, all glitter and glamour, ready to wow everyone at the party—it's that dazzling persona you switch on to impress others, not your most authentic-authentic self. Wearing the flashiest mask at the ball feels fun for a while, but when you get home you feel that much more let down by the person underneath it, not believing that you're inherently beautiful just as you are.

THE TOOLBOX OF THE SELF-ABANDONMENT CYCLE

So far, we've explored the way that shame prompts us to self-abandon—to cover up and leave behind those messy, imperfect, burdensome true selves in favor of Survival Selves that help us feel safe, included, and valued. But self-abandonment isn't a one-time thing—it's a cyclical relational dynamic. What I mean is that Emotional Outsourcing traps us in a cycle where our attempts to source safety, worth, and belonging from those around us leave us disappointed, that disappointment feels unsafe, and so we distance ourselves from the version of ourself who "caused" that disappointment. In other words, we self-abandon.

We Martyr ourselves or swoop in, Fixer to the rescue, expecting that the Survival Self personas we've adopted will ensure that we are valued, included, and safe. But that's not always what happens. Maybe that friend didn't actually love the way you told her she was stupid if she didn't dump her boyfriend, or they resent the way you always make decisions for them (and the subsequent guilt trips about how much you do for them). Maybe the people in your life don't feel as cared for, grateful, or happy as you expected them to. They don't shower you with the unconditional love and support you were longing for in exactly the way you wanted it when you wanted it. So you get upset because, let's be real with ourselves, love, we didn't really want to do all that extra stuff in the first place. Especially without the ego (read: safety) boost we expected and craved, it doesn't feel good to live at the ends of our ropes pretending it's all fine and we've got it together when we're exhausted and resentful.

Let's look at an example. My client Penelope had been feeling distant from her wife, Max, and wanted to do something that might resolve the tension building between them. She knew Max had had a rough week (corporate had decided to shutter one of their factories, and she had to break the news to more than a hundred workers) and thought that maybe the comforting smells of her favorite meal for Friday dinner might make her a little warmer. But Max barely acknowledged the effort. Penelope had spent hours in the kitchen, but she barely got a muted thank-you before Max started scrolling on her phone. Pen was angry. She felt dismissed, unappreciated—how could Max not recognize that she'd gone to all this effort! But the second that indignation reared its head, Penelope's inner critic was there to cut her down to size. *What, did you really think beef tibs and homemade injera would make her love you again?* it asked her scornfully. *It's not like it's even that hard to make. You're stupid to be mad about this; you'll just have to try harder.* Upset, she excused herself to "check on dessert," and in the kitchen, she busied herself with unnecessary tidying, unwittingly using these habitual cleaning tasks to avoid confronting Max or acknowledging her hurt feelings, even to herself really. Setting the sponge back in its holder, she realized it was probably her fault—the beef was a little overdone anyway—and it wasn't like anything she tried ever worked anyway.

See how that happens? The moment Penelope's attempt to connect wasn't met with the gratitude and enthusiasm she expected—when her partner didn't generate the feelings she was counting on to make her feel better—she turned that hurt inward. She invalidated her authentic reaction (disappointment, sadness) and self-abandoned, slipping back into the familiar thought patterns of the Scapegoat and Victim mind-sets she had seen modeled for her at home as a teenager.

Creating distance between our authentic self and our Survival Self is a core part of the self-abandonment cycle. Folks with Emotional Outsourcing develop a whole repertoire of well-worn strategies to maintain that separation—a self-abandonment toolbox, if you will. And while there are many ways to disconnect from the true self and slip into the false self that feels necessary for survival, there are three I see in my coaching clients *every single time*: buffering, ruminating, and overfunctioning. These three are the "how" of self-abandonment—the ways we suppress, override, or outright reject our authentic needs, feelings, beliefs, and experiences.

Buffering

Buffering is the undisputed most common and universal habit of Emotional Outsourcing in my clients. The concept of buffering was first written about in the 1970s by psychology researchers Sheldon Cohen and Thomas Wills,[7] who proposed that social support systems can act as a protective factor against the negative effects of stress. We're using the term differently now, referring to anything we do to numb or distract ourselves from our emotions, needs, and desires in an unconscious attempt to put a barrier between us and facing the discomfort associated with life and the rawness of our human experience. It often looks like doomscrolling, watching Netflix, overeating, overexercising, or overachieving instead of feeling our feelings,[8] but it can manifest in a thousand different ways. Gossip and complaining can serve as buffers against feelings of disappointment, jealousy, or sadness. Thought-terminating clichés like "It is what it is" or "Boys will be boys!" or "It'll all work out" shut down conversations before we have to delve into territory that asks us to examine what we are truly thinking or feeling. Procrastination, too, is a form of buffering: a temporary escape from the overwhelm of our to-do list, personal challenges, and our own perfectionist mandates about How Things Should Be Done.

This one's a shocker for many of my clients: Did you know that self-help "healing work" can actually be a buffer? Folks who jump from book to program to retreat to guru to spiritual practice to plant medicine and so on, never taking the time to *integrate* new learnings, not pausing long enough to do the work associated with any one of those practices, let alone *actually* be in touch with the pain and stuckness that prompted them to start this journey to begin with, are often buffering against something deep-deep, in my experience.

So you see, my darling, what constitutes buffering isn't so much the action itself, but whether we're doing it with presence or we're using it to put distance between ourselves and the real, embodied experiences of our lives.

We buffer to navigate the profound and frightening discomfort of exposing our true selves in a world that often seems (or very much is) unsafe for such vulnerability.[9] It's a protective mechanism, a way to shield our genuine desires, needs, and emotions from the judgment and expectations of the world around us[10]—exactly like we were conditioned to do.[11]

When we find ourselves reaching for a distraction—a glass of wine, another episode, buying things, completing tasks nobody asked us to—it's rarely a conscious choice. In fact, our tendency to buffer is exacerbated by societal and intergenerational patterns that have distanced us from our bodies, the earth, our communities, and a sense of true interdependence.[12] So, my love, I'm 100 percent serious when I say that your buffering, like all our other survival skills, needs to be celebrated if you ever want to release the grip it has on you. In fact, did you know that beating yourself up about buffering is, in fact, buffering against feeling sad about buffering by feeling bad about it?[13] Brains are wild, huh?

Ruminating

Speaking of brains, has yours ever kept you up into the wee hours replaying your Most Awkward Moments? Like the time your new crush asked what you do for fun, and instead of answering like a normal person, you panicked and said, "I'm really into, uh... organizing my pantry?" The second it left your mouth, you could see the confusion flash across their face. *Organizing your pantry? What the hell?! That's the best you could come up with?* Now, as you lie in bed, you're replaying every second, over and over, convinced they think you're the most boring human alive. Not just awkward—boring and tedious and dull and and and... And no matter how hard you try, your brain keeps whispering, *Yep, this is why you're still single.* Yeah, totally... me neither.

My love, the ruminating is *real* for us Emotional Outsourcing folks. Our brains love to loop endlessly through worries, regrets, and what-ifs. This isn't reflecting or self-examination; when we ruminate, our mind becomes a battlefield, and peace feels like a distant, unattainable dream as we scrutinize our experiences from every angle and then some.

We ruminate to try to make sense of our distress, believing (falsely) that by replaying situations or projecting our worst fears about ourselves onto others, we can find solutions or gain insight. My client Sophia was a master of this. Every night after she finished wiping down the kitchen, she sat alone at the dining room table, her mind racing with thoughts of the day's failures: a harsh word to her daughter, a dinner not quite perfect, a fleeting moment of longing for her own dreams, quickly suppressed. This nightly ritual, a quiet symphony of guilt and self-criticism, became

Sophia's secret burden, a testament to her distorted self-image and obsessive self-monitoring.

Rumination stems from the brain's tendency to prioritize negative information processing as a survival strategy, often leading to a persistent focus on perceived threats or unresolved issues.[14] When we ruminate, the prefrontal cortex is actively piecing together past experiences and projecting future outcomes, often as a way of trying to solve problems or prepare for potential challenges.[15] Some rumination takes the form of what I call "time traveling"—a kind of mental escapism where we get stuck living in the past, obsessively considering what has been or worrying about what could be, which takes us out of the present (and our ability to actually change our lives) in every way.

Overfunctioning

If you were a parentified child, had emotionally immature parents, or learned early on that love and care had to be earned, overfunctioning might feel all too familiar. It's the habit of taking on excessive responsibility and caretaking in relationships, often at the cost of your own well-being. When we don't feel emotionally or physically connected to our people, or when our true selves don't feel significant to them, we overextend—doing everything possible to prove we matter, desperately seeking connection in any way we can.

Our solution is to do the Very Mostest, attempting to outrun our fear that we're not good enough or ever doing enough—leaning *hard* on that sympathetic activation and riding the waves of cortisol and adrenaline as far as they'll take us before crashing, then dusting ourselves off, pounding another cup of coffee, and carrying on like it's nothing. Because it has to be—we're "fine," *remember?*

When we're mired in our Emotional Outsourcing habits, overfunctioning can, and usually does, show up in all aspects of our lives. My perfect snickerdoodle, *of course* you overfunction if you base your self-worth on the opinion of those around you and you believe that those people can only think well of you when you're keeping them happy, doing everything you're asked, anticipating what they'll need next, and so on, doing things for them they may not have even wanted you to do—so it's no wonder you resent them for not appreciating your labors enough. The shame of not being enough would be too much to bear, so you push down your authentic real self and do enough to convince anyone in a ten-mile radius that you are The Person Who Can Do Anything.

Sylvia was that go-to person at her office. Fresh out of college and eager to prove herself, she was always game to lend a hand or to take on another project, no matter the cost to her own well-being. Her reputation as endlessly dependable, while flattering, was a double-edged sword. Each yes was a desperate plea for validation, a silent scream for recognition that she mattered. As her workload grew, so did her sense of isolation, her days a blur of tasks completed in the hope of filling the void of unmet emotional needs. In this cycle of overextension, Sylvia lost more than time; she lost pieces of herself, and her youth, sacrificed at the altar of indispensability.

In overfunctioning, we continually put ourselves last and make decisions that require us to ignore or repress our own feelings. We overcompensate for our frustrations by doing things for others that they could so totally do for themselves, shoving down those (supposedly) inconvenient, rude, unwelcome, resentful parts of ourselves, holding them underneath the surface of our reality a little like holding a beach ball underwater. We overfunction and feel taken advantage of and let that resentment build and build and build until, just like that beach ball popping up out of the water when we just can't hold it anymore, it explodes outward, usually at our loved ones. Suddenly, it's us, not them, who are acting badly or being unreasonable (which lets the underfunctioning folks in our lives off the hook). We feel so guilty for raising our voice, for expressing our feelings and needs, for telling it like it is (or, okay, even throwing a pillow), that we're right back where we started: beating ourselves up for having needs and feelings, for daring to want mutuality and respect in our relationships. The shame is overwhelming, and we overcompensate by doing what we know how to do best and overfunctioning to hold our true selves at bay and keep those around us happy.

Overfunctioning isn't just a personal or relational habit—it's a deeply conditioned survival strategy, shaped by sociocultural forces that equate worth with output and reward self-sacrifice, especially for women and people from marginalized communities. In a world that prizes relentless productivity and expects certain groups to shoulder the emotional and physical burdens of others, overfunctioning becomes less of a choice and more of an expectation. The message is clear: Your value isn't in who you are, but in how much you can do—for your family, your workplace, your community. And when that belief is woven into the fabric of a society, it stops feeling like an external imposition and starts to feel like the natural order of things.

My client Claire kept the house running like a well-oiled machine—and her husband comfortably underfunctioning within it. Up before the sun, she packed lunches, answered work emails between flipping pancakes, made a mental note to grab her mother-in-law's prescription, and preemptively rescheduled her son's dentist appointment so it wouldn't interfere with her husband's golf game. He moved through the house unhurried, sipping his coffee, assuming things would get done because, well, they always did. When she finally sat down at the end of the day—after reminding him (again) to take the trash out—he sighed, stretched, and said, "You never just *relax*." And she almost laughed. *Relaxation* was a luxury afforded to those whose lives weren't held together by an endless to-do list, a lifetime of anticipating needs before they became problems, and a marriage where one person's ease was built on the other's exhaustion.

For women, especially, the expectation to be nurturing, capable, and endlessly available is often framed as a virtue—selflessness as an aspirational ideal. But beneath that glorification lies a systemic demand for overfunctioning, a push to prioritize others' needs at the cost of one's own. For many, particularly BIPOC folks and those in other marginalized communities, this pressure is compounded by the weight of systemic oppression, which insists that worthiness must be proven through relentless labor, caretaking, and an unwavering capacity to endure. Over time, these external pressures shape internal narratives, making overfunctioning feel less like a burden imposed from the outside and more like an unquestionable personal duty.

All this is to say, sweet one, self-abandon for long enough and you'll lose track of where you end and where anyone else starts, which is the root of so many quintessential Emotional Outsourcing relationship dynamics.

RELATIONSHIP CONSEQUENCES OF EMOTIONAL OUTSOURCING

So far, we've spent a lot of time looking at ourselves—the stories we learned growing up, how our nervous systems learned to react to keep us functional in the face of the overwhelming and threatening reality that we might not be loved and accepted just as we are. We've seen how shame leads us to abandon ourselves and adopt the oh-so-familiar tropes of folks living from codependent, people-pleasing, and perfectionist scripts. But as I said at the very beginning, Emotional Outsourcing is an inherently relational conundrum, and, my loves, it's time to look at how these components come together to impact our relationships.

Fundamentally, folks stuck in Emotional Outsourcing do not have a clear sense of self. This isn't about losing touch with our preferences; it's about a profound inauthenticity that seeps into every crevice of our lives, rendering us more as actors in someone else's play rather than the protagonists of our own stories. We are professional other-people-prioritizers—fawning and people-pleasing at all times, saying yes when we want to say no, and we have never heard of a boundary. (*What if they needed me? What if they feel upset if I say no? Better not . . .*)

When you stack it all up, it's really no surprise that emotional outsourcers end up in relationships where we feel, at best, invisible and underappreciated and, at worst, exploited and abused. You have been taught to move through life invalidating your own dignity and ignoring your needs, wants, emotions, and experience, and—painful as it feels to our tender hearts and yearning souls—you ended up in relationship roles and patterns that don't serve you. How could it be otherwise?

I need to be real with you, my love: these relationship dynamics we're about to explore? Well, you helped build them. I know it doesn't feel that way. But the reality is that by the time we are adults, we're so terrified of being wrong or bad or imperfect—of feeling the deathlike blows of rejection and shame—that we don't, and seemingly can't, take responsibility for our baloney. We blame everyone else because it would be just too existentially threatening to consider that maybe, just maybe, we were part of (and in some instances, okay, maybe even all of) the problem. We're too disconnected from our self to see how we're hurting ourselves and others because of the simple fact that we don't see ourselves as the main character. Life seemingly happens *to* us, not because of us.

As you learn more about these relationship patterns, I want you to offer yourself gentle accountability—with "gentle" as the operative word. Hold in mind your various romantic relationships (current and past), friendships, colleague dynamics, and so forth, and try to notice how each relationship challenge shows up for you, looking for patterns. Clarity requires grace—offer yourself the opportunity to understand, so that you can access that potential for change in the future. This is not an invitation to be cruel to you, but rather, to own your piece of this pie so you can change it up for the future.

Relationship Magical Realism

"Relationship magical realism" is the term I coined while teaching a relationship course back in 2014 to explain the fantastical ways in which folks with codependent, perfectionist, and people-pleasing tendencies focus on the potential of a relationship rather than its reality. It can apply to a friend, sibling, or work buddy as much as a romantic relationship, though it's often most pronounced in the latter. When we're engaged in relationship magical realism, we can't really see the red flags, those glaring warning signs of trouble, through the haze of wishful fantasy thinking and stories like "He says he wants to change" or "She doesn't seem to want to change, but I'll show her how amazing it would be if she did!" Meanwhile green flags, indicators of healthy relationship potential, are lost in the shadows of our own doubts and fear and just become something else to feel anxious about.

I've engaged in magical realism in most of my relationships. I was convinced I'd finally be the one to make them want to exercise, eat well, keep house the way I thought was right, or communicate the way I needed. I especially did this in my first marriage, where I thought I could change their lifelong habits of sedentary self-neglect, cruel communication, overdrinking, and chain-smoking. I took their counterfeit yeses to the bank and was surprised every time when my spouse hadn't changed one bit. Stuck in my Fixer ways, I convinced myself there was something I could do—so I poured my time, energy, emotional bandwidth, money, and resources into trying to shape them into the person I wanted them to be. The person they *claimed* they wanted to be but had no real interest in becoming. All so I could prove to myself that I was worthy of the love I craved from the kind of person I wanted it from . . . someone they clearly weren't and never wanted to be. Like so many of my clients, I was living under the belief that I had to show up unconditionally in my relationship—no expectations, no boundaries, no needs. Just endless giving. Codependent thought habits and self-sacrifice weren't just encouraged; they were the gold standard of marriage.

Thankfully, I can see now that I had it twisted. Love is, by definition, unconditional. If your affection, admiration, and respect for the person you love has conditions, that's not real love. That's something else, like manipulation or control. But relationships—the ways we choose to show up, connect, and share with one another—*need* conditions to thrive. Nobody gets to treat you however they please without consequence—without regard for your needs, desires, bodily autonomy, or what makes you feel loved. Choices have impact, and relationships aren't a free pass to disregard that. You get to decide what is and isn't okay, what is necessary, and what is a deal breaker if someone wants to be in relationship with you.* And this is what we forget in Emotional Outsourcing: that being with us is an amazing gift, and we don't just have to give ourselves away to anyone who wants us. Until we learn to set boundaries and advocate for ourselves in relationships—something that can feel like an existential threat to our nervous systems—we're likely to find ourselves stuck in romantic partnerships, friendships, and kinship relationships that are confusing, unsatisfying, and exploitative—conditional to the core.

Acting from Over-Responsibility

When we enter relationships from a place of codependent thinking, we have an unfortunate tendency to overstep boundaries by shouldering responsibility for everything and everyone.

---

* We often call these conditions boundaries. If that word gives you hives or makes you sweat just thinking about it, don't worry, I'll help you kitten-step your way through this in chapter 8. One piece at a time, my love.

That constant focus on managing, fixing, or controlling situations or emotions for others can lead us to neglect our own needs, feelings, and responsibilities.

Essentially, we feel more responsible to the (real or imagined!) needs and expectations of the folks around us than we do to ourselves. And how could we not, my little marigold? This is, after all, the very definition of Emotional Outsourcing: Uncertain of our own worth and the role we have in the lives of the people around us, we look to them for the validation we don't think we can give ourselves. We depend on their ease and happiness to soothe our dysregulated nervous systems, so we can't tolerate when others are stressed or distressed—it's too upsetting for our own nervous systems.

My client Andrea was notorious in her friend group for changing plans and rescheduling her life at the drop of a hat for others—the hat in this case being driving an hour to pick up lawn chairs from a store four towns over that her son mentioned maybe wanting (*Can't leave those sitting. What if my son needs them right away? I'll go to the doctor another time*), or dinner plans with a friend (*My husband's going to be home that night after all, so I'd better stay home and make dinner*), or being late to her first meeting at a new job because her colleague texted that *she* was running late to work (*Obviously, she won't have time for her usual coffee stop—and we all know how grumpy she is without coffee! I'll pop in and get her a latte to make sure she's good for the day*).

The problem isn't just that we're running ourselves ragged; it's that all those years of stuffing it down wear us down, and we begin to take it out on the people around us. Because we're constantly going out of our way and overextending ourselves for everyone else, when we don't get the immediate validation we're looking for, the cycle of self-abandonment activates in earnest. All those years of not feeling seen or appreciated start to bubble out sideways through resentment, irritability, annoyance, and passive aggression. Instead of focusing inward, understanding and owning our personal actions and consequences, we manifest our frustration in what's called *protest behavior.*[16] Frustrated but trapped in patterns that make asking for what we need feel impossible, our needs spill out sideways—we try to make the other person feel guilty, blaming and shaming them when we don't feel connected or validated. Statements like "I did everything for you last week even though I was so exhausted and burned out and overwhelmed. What do you mean you can't just show up for me right now in the exact way I need you to whether you want to or not?!" become constant refrains. We avoid making decisions because we fear we will make the wrong one, *and* we subconsciously push others into making our decisions for us so we have a fall guy in case it goes sideways. Sneaky, right?

Just like with overfunctioning, our tendency to shove it all down until we *explode* ensures that we remain caught in a dynamic where we feel that we're the bad guy (after all, we're the one acting out, yelling, and being "unreasonable"), and we feel so guilty about our behavior that we let the underfunctioner off the hook, taking on an even more outsized sense of responsibility in the relationship.

Acting from over-responsibility creates a dynamic where intrusiveness is mistaken for care and avoidance of self-accountability is normalized, leaving kids who grew up this way to think it's normal and acceptable for both them and future partners to evade responsibility.[17] Getting vulnerable again here, this was very much the dynamic in my abusive first marriage. I was a high-achieving overfunctioner, deep in my own Emotional Outsourcing, and had been doing extra chores and household work since I was in elementary school in an attempt to regulate my nervous system through doing, and as a way to source safety, validation, and attachment externally*—which is all a small kiddo really

* On average, the development of the ability to source feelings of safety, validation, approval, and self-regulation from within tends to become more pronounced during the

can do, developmentally speaking.[18] So of course I found a partner (a wealthy spoiled child of a major Martyr mom) who was only too happy to declare that they didn't have to make the bed, do the laundry or dishes, cook or do grocery shopping, or do any emotional labor—ever, and I was a nag and a bitch for asking them to. They didn't have to be responsible because I was there to be over-responsible for them—just like their mother had been their whole life, and, *oof*, did it feel terrible to be treated like a servant all those years, while the gaslighting kept me stuck in it, convinced by them that I was the one and only problem.

So many of us living in Emotional Outsourcing either find partners who don't want to participate in an interdependent reciprocal relationship, or overfunction to the point that, even if they came into the relationship wanting to do their part, they eventually stop—it's easier to just let you be a whirlwind of doing than to actually do anything for themselves, because that will displease you, and no one wants that. Same goes for friends and jobs too, my love. Over-givers have an uncanny ability to find the over-takers, and most people aren't going to work too hard convincing you to do less for them.

As the person living from Emotional Outsourcing continues to sacrifice their needs, desires, and well-being, driven by the shame-based belief that their value lies solely in their ability to care for others, they put more and more of their sense of value in their ability to sustain unfulfilling and exhausting relationships. And here's the kicker: In this cycle of overfunctioning, we don't realize that we are blocking ourselves from receiving love, care, kindness, and support—the very things we've been trying to manufacture. Receiving can feel strange, uncomfortable, and even scary when we're not used to it, so we push it away and do it

---

adolescent years, which typically range from ages twelve to eighteen. This is a general guideline, and individual variations are significant.

all ourselves to avoid that feeling of unease. It feels like care can't come without strings, like it's bound to be "used against us," and in shielding ourselves from potential future harms, we block ourselves from being cared for now.

Terrible Communication

Let's be honest with ourselves, lovelies: We're lousy communicators. We didn't get much practice speaking directly and kindly, didn't have modeling of speaking up for ourselves, asking things of others who would actually like to say yes or even hear us, or having honest conversations, so we frequently resort to indirect remarks, critiques, and passive aggression instead of being direct. We grumble, complain, find fault in everything, and reject *every* offer of help. A glass of water after crossing the Sahara on foot? "Oh no, I'm fine." Help schlepping a thousand bags of groceries in from the car in one go? "Nope, I've got it." Your friend holds space for you to talk about the rough time you've been having since your mom passed. "Oh, thank you, but, yeah—I'm okay, I'm fine." And don't you dare try to give a gal a thoughtful present! She won't begin to even know how to start to accept it!

For most of us, this pattern is deeply rooted in a profound fear of both conflict and connection—each one tangled up with vulnerability in our kiddo minds and bodies. Conflict, obviously, constitutes failure in a world where your job is to keep everyone happy with you at all times. And vulnerability? That requires feelings that are just too scary and too challenging to tap into... they've been frozen for too long.

Without the skills or capacity to communicate authentically, we develop the unfortunate habit of expecting that others can and should read our minds the way we always try to read theirs. When our unspoken expectations aren't met, we shame ourselves, reinforcing that it's dumb and stupid to want anything or to need anyone. Once again, the pressure of not having expressed our true feelings builds, resentment seethes beneath the surface, and eventually we boil over into another round of the self-abandonment cycle, or explode on the nearest available human.

Further complicating our communication is our tendency to project onto other people. Projection happens when you treat the now like the past, as though a movie projector were shining the stories of things and people that were no darn good onto people and things in your present moment. And, *wow*, does it make life harder than it needs to be. When we project, we're stuck watching a rerun of an old script, where the cast, plot, and drama are all our own creations—our fears, assumptions, and insecurities playing the lead roles. This habit doesn't just skew our perception; it effectively derails any chance of true understanding, as we've already written our role *and* theirs before they've had a chance to speak. So, we respond to what we imagined they meant rather than what they actually said, turning even neutral exchanges into battlegrounds we're fighting from both sides.

Projection is part of the reason we so masterfully anticipate criticism or rejection where there might be none. It sounds like a counterintuitive defense mechanism, but by projecting our own fear, worry, and insecurity outward, we believe we're insulated from experiencing those painful feelings directly because we pre-felt them in a way.[19] But, oh boy, does it make it hard to communicate! People who project (aka pretty much everyone living in Emotional Outsourcing) rarely hear what other people *actually* say, filtering it, instead, through the lens of what they expected to hear based on past experience, their own fears and insecurities, or how they're feeling in the moment. It's that moment when your partner asks if there's any more toothpaste and you jump down their throat, defensively protesting that it shouldn't always have to be your responsibility to keep everything stocked and know where everything is . . . but they were actually just asking because they were about to head to the store. It's when your mom sighs after a long day, and you immediately assume she's annoyed with *you*, even though she hasn't said a word about it. It's when a friend takes a little longer to reply to a text, and your brain fills in the silence with *They're mad at me. I must have said something wrong.*

The final nail in our communication coffin has to do with boundaries. Short version? We don't have 'em. We've already seen how losing track of where you end and where others begin can lead to intrusiveness, but it goes beyond that to color moments of potential connection. In essence, we don't know how to have compassion for folks without trying to fix them. We think that solutions and solidarity are the same thing because that's what was shown to us. For example, when Jo's cousins were discussing the challenges of parenting teenagers, she couldn't resist the urge to chime in with her own (very unsolicited) advice. "You really should set firmer boundaries," she interjected confidently, launching into a detailed account of how she managed her own children, sending podcast episodes and recommending the books that they should read. Her relatives exchanged polite but slightly strained smiles—rather than closeness, Jo's insistent recommendations and lack of boundaries only created more distance. The irony . . .

Reenactment

Reenactment, from a nervous system perspective,[20] is when we unconsciously re-create and relive past experiences—especially those rooted in trauma or significant emotional events—in an attempt to resolve what was left unresolved. We repeat familiar scripts, take familiar actions, and hope, this time, for a different, more healing outcome.[21] This is known as repetition compulsion, and it can be subtle, often masked as instinctive reactions to certain stimuli (like if you only got praise as a kid when you got a gold star, having to do a work presentation might make you anxious or stressed), or it can be more overt, significantly influencing our life choices and interpersonal dynamics—such as whom you choose as your romantic partner.[22]

This process of replaying our childhood relationships in adulthood is so very common, my love. Ask any therapist and they'd be only too happy to confirm that almost every person they see is reenacting something. Remember how your nervous system is always trying its darndest to take care of you? Reenactment is your subconscious attempt to get in adulthood what you didn't get, and needed, as a kid. For folks who grew up with codependent, people-pleasing, and perfectionist scripts, this often means that we show up in our relationships as over-givers seeking to rebalance the proverbial scales of give and get, hoping that this time (this time!) we shall give our all and get our due: unconditional, fathomless appreciation and validation, often for doing important things, but also for doing things that nobody at all, like 0.00 percent of people, asked us to do.

The problem is that even though it doesn't usually work, our nervous systems prefer a comfortable hell to an unknown heaven,* which means that we will tend to do the same thing over and over again even when it sucks, effectively because it hasn't gotten us killed yet, which our nervous system sees as a win overall (the not-dead-yet part).

In Emotional Outsourcing, reenactment can keep us feeling stuck in a cycle where we continually seek approval and validation, mirroring early life experiences where these behaviors were often necessary for acceptance and emotional survival. These habits, deeply ingrained in our neurobiological wiring, perpetuate a loop of behaviors that might feel safe but are ultimately counterproductive to our emotional and psychological well-being.[23]

I've heard this story over and over from clients over the last decade: "I hate this job/marriage/date/whatever" and "I'm stuck and can't get out," and often that's a reenactment talking. This is a

---

* This statement is often attributed to the philosopher and psychologist Carl Jung; however, we have no solid proof that he was the first dude to say it, so do with that what you will.

story that comes up because, in a way, you *can't* get out yet—not until you're able to recognize what's going on in your mind and body and make the subconscious conscious, as it were. Your nervous system is looking for a reason to stop doing what it's doing, my love. And while reenactment is unlikely to break the self-abandonment cycle that kept you safe all these years, what *does* shift it is intentional, deliberate choiceful, science-backed, loving intervention.

~

My love, it's time to reclaim your true self. You are enough, and you deserve to know as deeply and immutably as I do that you are worthy and lovable and good, just for being who you really are. I want you to form relationships where you can give lovingly from a full cup, not because you fear that you won't be loved if you don't overfunction to the point of exhaustion. I want so much for you to create and believe new stories about yourself, restore access to your body so you're not living from the neck up, learn new patterns of thinking, and create boundaries that help you say, "Me first, you second, us together, with love." You deserve to know where you stop and others begin, and to step into new relationship patterns from a space of mutual support, mutual respect, and mutual trust. To do that, we're going to make some big changes. Are you ready, my love? Be gentle, go slow, and stick with it. And, when you're ready, turn the page to start a new chapter—of this book, sure, and most of all, of your life.

JOURNAL PROMPTS
WORKING WITH SHAME, SELF-ABANDONMENT, AND RELATIONSHIP PATTERNS

I know how overwhelming it can feel to examine our own behaviors and relationship patterns. Just noticing the chasm between the person you've stepped into and the real, authentic you can feel like touching a live wire. As always, I want you to go slow as you approach these questions. Give yourself space to express your observations and feelings—your journal and your journey are *yours*. I promise there is never any shame in getting honest with yourself.

1. When I feel shame, how do I know that's what I'm feeling (e.g., a familiar thought or voice, a physical sensation)?

   ....

   ....

   ....

2. In what circumstances do I feel the most shame? Why might that be?

   ....

   ....

   ....

3. When I hold on to shame, what do I think I'm protecting myself from? What do I gain from shaming myself?

   ....

   ....

   ....

4. When do I shame others? What does that do for me ('cause it's doing something or you wouldn't be doing it!)?

....

....

....

5. What Survival Self resonated most for me? What feels familiar about it? (I.e., what feels reminiscent of what I learned with my family of origin?)

....

....

....

6. What thoughts and feelings are most uncomfortable for me to sit with? What do I believe about myself when those thoughts/emotions come up?

....

....

....

7. Write down three activities that you engage in as buffers. For each activity, answer these questions:

....

   - What might I be avoiding by doing this?

....

....

....

- What is going on in my mind right before I do this? What sensations do I notice in my body?

....

....

....

- What advantage might there be to feeling this feeling, or engaging with that thought?

....

....

....

8. Where am I not taking responsibility for my actions in my relationships? Where am I taking responsibility?

....

....

....

9. Think about a recent time you felt frustrated in a relationship. With loving accountability, ask yourself whether, and to what extent, relationship magical realism, over-responsibility/overfunctioning, and/or your communication have played a role in that situation.

....

....

....

10. What do you think you're reenacting with your romantic partner (past or present)? What do you think you needed (or needed more of) in childhood that you're trying to source from your current relationships? Do you think that's something you're likely to experience if you continue acting, thinking, and experiencing the world in the same ways you are currently?

Part 2

Becoming Interdependent

Chapter 5

Be the Cake

It's time, my glorious *mariposas*: We're finally stepping into part 2, where you're going to learn the strategies and tools you need to begin to shift your sense of self, your nervous system, your thoughts, and your relationships so that you can step into interdependence—that mutual, reciprocal way of relating that honors self-trust first, connection second, and love as the foundation.

You've already begun the hard work of seeing yourself clearly, and by now you are familiar with the way suboptimal attunement from your caregivers (compounded by the oppressive systems that govern our world) stressed your nervous system and led you to believe that safety, self-worth, and belonging were available to you only if you behaved in ways that were accepted by the people around you—shaming yourself out of your authentic needs and feelings until you eventually abandoned your sense of self altogether and learned to relate to your world through Emotional Outsourcing. And, *oof!* My love! That is so much for little you to have handled!

By this point in your adult life I'm willing to bet that you're so fully accustomed to focusing your attention and energy outward—as one living from Emotional Outsourcing is so very likely to do—that you may not even realize that's what you're doing when you feed everyone else but don't eat, when you get everyone else ready but don't take time to shower (while making sure to complain about how long-suffering you are because it doesn't count if others don't know you're suffering for them, right?), when you acquiesce constantly and don't even know what you're feeling, wanting, or needing. When we live from our false selves and buffer against our authenticity in an effort to get by without exploding, we lose track of who we are and what matters to us—we can't see ourselves. We aren't present or regulated so we're stuck living in old patterns—because how else *could* we be living?

And in sacrificing so much of yourself—your energy, time, attention, desires, needs—you became a Giving Tree of sorts, giving and giving until there was nothing left that was you.

The start of our healing process looks like interrupting the self-blame and self-abandonment cycle by reclaiming our sense of self. This means prioritizing our own needs, pursuing personal interests, and cultivating a sense of self that is independent of relationships where codependent living rules, and we're going to spend the rest of this chapter focusing on just that: remedies that can help you give yourself center stage in your own life, honoring what has been, and learning how to begin to shift for the future.

It may feel selfish at first, but I promise it's only self-*ish*. When you've lived your life for other people for as long as you have, sweet butternut blossom, you need to start this journey toward authenticity, interdependence, and joy by reclaiming who you are—a person who knows their own mind, and who knows they are worthy of kindness, attention, and support. A person who knows in their bones that they're the whole enchilada—or, as I like to teach my students, the cake.

Ground Rules: The Wisdom of Kitten Steps

My love, I have only one ask of you as you start making changes to end those Emotional Outsourcing habits: I want to invite you to take kitten steps. You've probably heard others extol the virtues of baby steps, but frankly, I've found through my decade plus in coaching that baby steps can be way too big and overwhelming as a starting place. I mean, a baby's foot is, on average, three inches long—that's a third the size of your adult human foot![1] My love-bug, changing 30 percent of your life in one fell swoop as a starting place is just not going to set you up for success, but rather, it will set you up to wobble trying to change it all, New Year's resolution–style, and fall down on your perfect snout! To see sustainable, long-term change, you need to let your nervous system get used to small changes before ramping it up, and a newborn kitten's paw is quite small indeed—so take that size step!

With love, we're not going to do what our perfectionist habits yearn to and go from couch to CrossFit in one week, or try out boundaries for the very first time by starting with your emotionally unavailable parent. Focus on moving forward one set of wee, precious toe beans at a time. I promise, the slower you go, the farther your efforts will take you (and the less your nervous system will freak out).

GETTING TO SELF-COMPASSION

Be honest, my lovely one: How many times have you heard that term and kind of rushed on by it? I know it took me years to truly understand what it means to have compassion for myself. When we've been conditioned (as we have in Emotional Outsourcing) to stuff down our true feelings and beliefs and measure our worth by everyone else's measuring sticks, it can be hard to show ourselves understanding, love, and care. When that vicious inner critic is in the driver's seat pulling on your hair and reminding you that your house is a mess (which means you've failed) and you need to lose five pounds (major fail, you!) and you're behind on your to-do list (ugh—seriously? you're the worst) and that gal on Instagram's closet is like *way* more organized than yours (which, again, makes you terrible) and why aren't you meal prepping right (answer: because you're worthless), it can feel downright impossible to bring self-compassion in. I know from my own experience how hard it was to see my own pain and attend to it deeply and with care—the way I so often (from my own codependent framework) would rush to attend the pain of others. Instead, we pile it on ourselves as though that would actually do anything other than keep us spinning in self-recrimination, indecision, and overwhelm.

For example, during a rare moment of quiet reflection, Leslie found herself replaying the argument she had with her husband, Gerard, the night before. It had started over something trivial—she had forgotten to pick up his dry cleaning, which he needed for an important meeting. His frustration was understandable, but Leslie's reaction to her mistake was disproportionate. She berated herself relentlessly, a tirade of self-criticism: *How could I be so careless? I'm ruining his career and this marriage. Why can't I ever do anything right?!* See how much deeper and more hurtful those self-inflicted jabs are than the thing that actually happened, my love? Gerard was only low-grade annoyed, yet Leslie took it to a 47 on a 1–10 scale out of habit, unintentionally negating his feelings by making it all about her. She was so cruel to herself that the sheer intensity of it overwhelmed her, leaving her unable to actually do anything to help. All she could do was sit in the swamp of her own lousy self-regard.

Buddhists call what Leslie did "shooting the second arrow." It goes like this: Life is gonna get lifey sometimes and send an arrow our way, like, you effed up a work call, an event you'd been looking forward to gets rained out, your partner forgot your anniversary, or you got sick right before a vacation and spent that precious PTO languishing on your couch instead of chillin' beachside. The original thing that sucks happened because life. That's the first arrow. When we chew ourselves out, ruminate on our mistakes and failures, or shame ourselves for not being able to do it all perfectly all the time, well, my love, that's suffering that we have brought on ourselves. Life shot the first arrow, but we shot the second one into our own tender hearts, and then sometimes we shoot the third arrow when we get mad at ourselves for making ourselves feel bad about messing up! It's not necessary or helpful, and so often it feels like it happens so quickly we don't even realize we're doing it.

Self-criticism activates the body's stress response (ye ol' fight or flight/sympathetic), leading to a cascade of physiological changes—increased heart rate, a spike in adrenaline, and a state of heightened arousal,[2] which means you're more freaked out than the moment calls for. These reactions are not just fleeting emotional states; they are embodied experiences that impact our physical health. Moreover, from a neuroscience perspective, activating the second arrow can reinforce harmful, negative neural pathways or habitual ways of thinking. The brain is malleable, adapting to our habitual thoughts and emotions. When we repeatedly engage in self-criticism, we strengthen the neural networks associated with these meanie-pants patterns, making them more likely to be our default response in the future.[3]

I am sorry to report that, despite years of searching, I have yet to find a magic switch that will flip us from a hard-won black belt in Emotional Outsourcing to never again looking for our sense of self, self-worth, safety, and belonging anywhere except inside ourselves. You've heard me say it before, my eager perfectionist bunny, and I'm going to say it again: Healing takes time. It's not linear. And it requires patience and that we stop being so darn mean to ourselves.

Many of us grew up believing that self-flagellating is the way to change, so we throw ourselves into the deep end of "self-improvement" without knowing how to tread water. I can't tell you how many clients have shared that, before we started working together, they tried to adopt a rigid meditation or work-out schedule that felt more punishing than peaceful, dove into intense personal development workshops without adequate emotional or nervous system support, or relentlessly journaled every perceived flaw in the name of "self-awareness."

Any attempt at change becomes a self-fulfilling prophecy: We set the bar so impossibly high that we're destined to fail. Then, when we do (drum roll please) it's second arrow time! We blame and shame ourselves so ferociously that we inadvertently reinforce our beliefs that we're inherently broken and not enough—never worthy of living a life with ease and good things.

Self-compassion is the armor we have against these second arrows.

We express compassion for ourselves when we show ourselves support, rather than cutting ourselves down when we make a mistake. We offer grace when we're facing life challenges instead of berating ourselves for not just magically being "better." Where we might normally criticize ourselves and belabor our shortcomings, self-compassion means seeing yourself in your full humanity—limitations and all—with acceptance and love rooted in an understanding of both societal conditioning and science.[4] It's the difference between thinking *Why am I such a lazy f*ck?!* and *Maybe it's not a problem if the dishes aren't done right now. I can do them later.* Self-compassion is the grace between *I should be able to do this by now! I'm so permaeffed that I'll never be able to be different and I'm going to be exhausted and stupid and alone forever* and *I'm trying to learn something hard and new, and I'm not always going to get it right.*

You can't hate yourself into positive change, love. I'm gonna say that over and over. (And maybe someone put it on a T-shirt, please!) Self-criticism and internalized negativity only serve to create a state of paralysis or avoidance and churn up a ton of nervous system dysregulation. When we're caught in the loop of self-criticism, our nervous system perceives threat, keeping us stuck in survival states—fight, flight, freeze, or fawn—rather than engaging the parts of the brain needed for learning, growth, and change. Instead of motivating us, harsh self-talk activates shame, which research shows decreases problem-solving abilities and self-efficacy. In contrast, self-compassion fosters neuroplasticity, emotional regulation, and the psychological safety necessary to take accountability and shift behaviors. In other words, self-criticism doesn't make us better—it keeps us trapped. When we're caught in the loop of self-criticism, we're less likely to take constructive action or learn from our mistakes. Instead, we become mired in a state of self-defeating rumination ('cause we're all up in that limbic system), and that self-blame only serves to keep us at arm's length from ourselves. I mean, it makes sense: Why would we want to know and care for a person we don't even like?![5] Meanwhile, the patriarchy and white-settler colonialism win time and again when we spend our limited time and energy beating ourselves up instead of naming the real problems and working to address them. Makes sense why they work so hard to keep us women, BIPOC folks, and others in marginalized bodies beating ourselves up, right?!

Kitten Step: "Of Course I Did!"

It's not uncommon for the perfectionist scripts we learned in childhood or adolescence to give birth to a pretty wicked inner critic. The lash of shame comes fast, furious, and painful when we don't get something exactly right. And for those of us who've relied on Emotional Outsourcing to survive, self-compassion can feel like weakness, excuse-making, or even something we don't deserve—none of which feel desirable or safe. I hear from clients that expressing self-compassion feels about as comfortable and possible as walking to the moon. And, hey, I get it.

When I was deepest in my own Emotional Outsourcing, the idea of cutting myself even the teensiest bit of slack was unthinkable. Tired? Too bad, I have errands and work to do. Headache or tummy ache? Too bad, you have patients to see. *Who do you think you are that you get a break? How could you be so selfish? Don't you know they'll leave if you're not perfect enough? Don't be such an eff-up!* my inner critic berated me. I was unfailingly kind, generous, and encouraging to the people around me... but showing myself even a smidge of the kindness I gave others? Fuggedaboutit. Why would I show compassion to myself? Why would I be nice to a dog that bites? What has it done to earn my kindness lately? It's a bad dog.

When we grow up in homes with emotionally immature caregivers—as I and so many of my clients did—we don't often have great models for self-compassion. More often than not, apologies and accountability are nonexistent. Child—you didn't *make* a mistake. You *were* the mistake. You didn't break a plate; you were a disappointment, or for some of my clients, a clumsy little effup. Dad didn't hurt your feelings; you're just too sensitive. You didn't (unavoidably) catch your sister's cold; you're a burden who ruined the whole weekend because someone had to stay home and take care of you—and taking care of you is not what they want to be doing; you're just adding to "all the ways I suffer for you children." Being seen for all my faults and foibles hadn't gone well for me in the past, so why would self-compassion, which, by definition, requires us to see ourselves in our full warts-and-all humanity, feel safe? No way. No how. No, thank you. So I came to believe that I had to earn compassion like I had to earn everything else: by being perfect and people-pleasing and never resting and constantly giving and doing and and and...

Folks with Emotional Outsourcing habits grow up walking a tightrope of perfection, all too aware that with just one misstep we'll fall to our (psychological and/or social) deaths—unlovable, useless, unworthy, and unwelcome forever. Shame is our gondolier's pole, the thing we grip tightly to keep ourselves feeling steady as we navigate precarious waters, using all our might to somehow push our way forward. And no matter how much it hurts to hold, when our sense of self is built on such unstable foundations, it can feel too risky to let go of the shame that's kept us upright for so many years. What if we tip? What if we sink? Trading shame for self-compassion is challenging, my love, so we're going to take a kitten step in the form of a simple phrase: "Of course I did."

Think of this phrase as your training wheels—a way to ease toward self-compassion and self-acceptance by cutting your self-judgment off at the knees. You see, when we say, "Of course I did!" we are working to see ourselves in context. You're not an idiot who can't remember anything; you were overwhelmed and multitasking as per usual, so *of course* you forgot to grab Cheerios at the store—that's what happens when we live in our Emotional Outsourcing survival skills. You aren't a spineless enabler who's wasting their time, but you *did* bail out your friend when they didn't plan ahead and needed a last-minute ride to the airport, because *of course you did*. You aren't a doormat, but you *did* say yes when you meant no when you got worried that maybe your boss wouldn't be happy to hear about your workload again, because *of course you did—you chronically and habitually source your sense of worth, safety, and belonging from everyone and everything outside yourself, to your deep and wild detriment because that's what you were taught would keep you safe.*

My kitten, let's be real: How could it be otherwise? The survival skills you learned and entrained into your nervous system are not failures. You are who you were trained to be. Remind yourself as many times as you need to that Emotional Outsourcing is the natural, normal, adaptive, *wise* way that your body and brain knew to keep you safe, and of course behaving this way says nothing about your character or who you actually are. *Of course* you put everyone and everything ahead of yourself and went out of your way for them, again, and then got resentful when they didn't seem particularly grateful. You aren't alone, and you came by those codependent, perfectionist, people-pleasing habits rightly.

And—instead of beating yourself up as a way to buffer against the grief, frustration, or disappointment you're really feeling when you notice your own Emotional Outsourcing patterns more closely, I invite you to acknowledge the bigger picture of your experience with a *loving* "Of course I did!" (which of course is the first step on the pathway to "Of course I used to").

Doubling down on shame, self-blame, second arrows, and triggering the self-abandonment cycle will not serve you as you continue this journey. As they say, "What got you here won't get you there," and I'd like to challenge you to take that kitten step and try on "Of course I did!" the next time you notice your inner critic winding up. Self-compassion isn't letting yourself off the hook. Rather, compassion allows you to take responsibility for your life, see what's yours to change, take steps to address that, and let the rest go. (Oh, and if you still harbor a fear that actually letting that inner critic ease up even a teensy bit would be a catastrophic mistake and doom you to a worthless, lonely life... well, my love, of course you do. It's okay. Take it one kitten step at a time.)

BE YOUR OWN WATCHER

As folks who live from Emotional Outsourcing habits, we are extremely talented at noticing and rationalizing (especially when it comes to other people's lousy behavior). You read people's emotions like it's the weather report, vigilant to any and all changes. You anticipate everyone's needs to reduce the risk of conflict, disagreement, or discomfort. You know exactly where society drew the line and do your utmost to stay at least three steps back to ensure your safety.

What we are not so great at noticing, my turtledove, is what's going on inside of our selves. In order to shift our experience of life, a vital first step is cultivating self-awareness, also known as being your own Watcher. In becoming your own Watcher, you shift from seeing yourself through the fun-house mirror of other people's opinions and reactions to noticing what's really going on inside your own mind and heart.

Perfectionists, people-pleasers, and all those with nervous system dysregulation, please take note that I did *not* invite you to become your own surveiller or judge! Your goal is not to scrutinize every detail of your existence and become even more hypervigilant to whether you're doing it "right." To be frank, those Emotional Outsourcing habits make sure we do plenty of judging and ruminating as is. The Watcher, by contrast, is responsible for observing your thoughts, feelings, projections, and behaviors *without* judgment.

Your Watcher knows that you have feelings, but *you* are not those feelings. Same with your thoughts and actions. With the removed curiosity of an academic on safari, your Watcher is there to notice patterns and bring your attention to your own experience. Building strong self-awareness often takes the form of something called *embodied insight*, which is a fancy way to explain the difference between recognizing a feeling intellectually and actually feeling it in your body and connecting those sensations to what's happening in your mind and environment. It's the difference between knowing that you feel overlooked and being fully present to the feeling of your hands trembling with righteous indignation. By raising your awareness of these physical cues and sensations, you can build your understanding of what leads to what within you, increasing your capacity and making you better equipped to navigate situations and respond with self-compassion.

Kitten Step: What Am I Feeling Right Now?

Let's try this out together, my love. I'll invite you to close your eyes and ask yourself two questions: (1) What am I feeling right now in this exact moment? and (2) where am I feeling that in my body? It may be tricky to discern at first, but as you step more and more into the role of your Watcher, you'll be able to check in with yourself and observe your thoughts, feelings, and habits fluently. Can't feel anything? No biggie. Try again later!

As you step into the role of Watcher, I recommend that you start by spending ten minutes each day in self-reflection to gain awareness of your emotions and feelings.* This could take the form of mindfulness meditation, journaling to notice your emotions (not just report what you did that day!), or dedicating five minutes a day to ask yourself some getting-to-know-you questions of yourself like it's the first day of summer camp. Don't complicate it or make it daunting, you silly goose! Keep it chill, light, and easy. The goal is to create opportunities to get to know yourself in a new way. However you want to structure your practice, I encourage you to start by asking questions like these:

* While emotions originate in the body, feelings are how we consciously experience and describe them. The somatic experience of both happens through interoception (our body's ability to sense its internal state), mediated by the vagus nerve and insular cortex.

- What emotions am I feeling right now?
- Where am I feeling this in my body?
- Are there any emotions I'm trying to avoid right now?
- How can I give the parts of me feeling those emotions love and care right now?

The more self-awareness you develop, the better you'll know what survival styles you're rocking in different moments and with different people, when you're buffering, when you're presenting a false self, when you're projecting your own stories and anxieties onto someone else, and so on. With time and practice, you can start to act on that information, deciding how you want to be and intervening lovingly for yourself, instead of just going along for the ride. Awareness itself is incredibly healing, so don't sleep on this part.

HAVE YOUR OWN BACK

Our Emotional Outsourcing habits have taught us that our choices, feelings, needs, and wants are valid only if other folks say so. In the long run, healing from Emotional Outsourcing means we have two choices: We can stand up for ourselves when needed, or—better yet—we can be unbothered and can let other people have their own thoughts and feelings without making them mean any thing about us as people. To start living from our true selves, we need to feel safe. In essence, we need to know that someone's got our back—and, my love, that "someone" gets to be you first and foremost.

When you have your own back, you know intrinsically, deeply, and without a doubt that you can be trusted to take care of yourself, because you evidence that to you all the time in big and kitten-sized ways. Most of us who grow up with Emotional Outsourcing habits have spent so long neglecting our basic biological impulses, our needs for nutrition, rest, solitude, even hygiene or medical care, that our brain has adopted the story that "I fail at self-care." We believe that we are no good at taking care of ourselves; ergo, we're not to be trusted to make decisions for ourselves or to know what's best for us—never mind the fact that we are excellent at taking care of everyone else and assume we know what's best for them.

I see this self-doubt and fear so often in my clients. They don't feel that they can make positive choices for their own lives (or even know what choices *are* positive) without external input. After years of silencing their inner voice, they can't feel the compass inside them pointing the way, they are no longer their own North Star. My client Christine struggled with this every time she set a goal. She'd identify something she wanted for herself—for example, a 5K she'd always dreamed of running—and in the same breath undercut that desire, saying things like "What if I'm the slowest person out there and make a fool of myself? My friend has gotten really into strength training lately—should I be doing that instead? Is a 5K even long enough to be a worthy goal? I know so many people training for marathons. Is this a stupid goal? Should I be trying harder? What do I know about training anyway? I'm a couch potato and I don't even have the right shoes. What if running hurts my knees?" She felt the familiar breeze of her helicopter mom hovering within her own psyche, ready to chime in with training plans and opinions about which races are best, along with opinions about this choice that make Christine doubt herself even more. It didn't take long before Christine felt so lost and overwhelmed that she lost sight of her desire and scrapped the whole project.

If little you didn't get the attunement you needed to feel safe and valued, you understandably started to doubt whether the grown-ups in your life could be trusted to take care of you. Your wise kiddo mind assumed it was all your fault and started distrusting and doubting yourself, too, and allathat is held in us as what many thought leaders such as psychologists John Bradshaw and Alice Miller and Buddhist monk Thich Nhat Hanh refer to as our inner child. As adults, our inner children (I see us as having many inner children, versus the common singular "inner child") continue to carry those unmet needs, wounds, traumas, and unresolved issues from childhood until we actively work to heal and release them.[6]

There are whole books written about inner child work, and for good reason. Getting to know our younger selves is a vital part of all journeys to heal, grow, and meet ourselves more deeply. I want to be clear that this work can be an adventure unto itself; however, for our purposes in rewiring Emotional Outsourcing, what I want to invite you to tap into is the way that these young parts of us persist today and, if we're not aware of their stories and their needs, can dictate how we show up in dating, work, parenting—every aspect of our lives, without our even realizing it. Whether they're loud and rowdy or quiet and scared, our inner children hold the stories we learned growing up that we didn't have the capacity to process then, and they impose their beliefs and fears on our adult lives. Without ever knowing it, so many of us are being driven by the wants, needs, and fears of our inner kiddos because (metaphorically speaking) there's a four-year-old trapped in your body throwing a tantrum to get your attention, believing that if they don't drive the bus of your adult life, something terrible will definitely happen.

Having coached thousands of people, I've come to believe that the farther your adult self leans into the codependent, people-pleasing, and perfectionist habits that once kept you safe, the less attuned you are to your own inner world. Desperate to get our attention, the kiddos yell louder, asserting needs that feel too dangerous to meet. True to our once-self-protective self-abandoning habits, we buffer, ruminate, overfunction, and turn away from ourselves, only proving to those young parts that *we* are now the adult who cannot be trusted to take care of us. Ouch.

Rebuilding self-trust means becoming the loving guardians our inner children need. The process is often referred to as "reparenting," but I think of it more broadly as an opportunity to give ourselves the love, attunement, compassion, and care we didn't get as children—not just to "parent" ourselves but to be the loving guardians our tender kiddo hearts really needed to protect and unconditionally love them.

Connecting with and becoming your own most loving guardian means knowing that *you* are the authority on your life, needs, values, and priorities, and therefore *you* are best positioned to call the shots in your own life, including where you put your focus and spend your time, energy, and resources. The more you take the time to attune to the needs of your inner children and show up to meet those needs with love as the guardian they needed, the more you reinforce the belief that "I matter to me, and I can be depended on to take care of me. Always. No matter what," and the more you solidify your unshakable self-trust.

Kitten Step: How Old Am I Right Now?

Inner child work is a beautiful and often complex process that can be started with a simple and loving question: How old am I being? How old is the part of me thinking, feeling, acting, in this moment? When we feel upset and dysregulated, it's often because a younger part of us is trying to protect or defend us, using the skills they have, given their age. So, the next time you feel upset or stirred up, sad without an obvious explanation, or angry at something you have no control over, having a big or too-small reaction, I want you to pause and ask yourself, *How old do I feel right now? How old is the part of me that's reacting so strongly to this situation?* Without judgment!

Are you whining and taking it personally like a four-year-old? Are you stomping your foot like a six-year-old?

Complaining and judging like a thirteen-year-old?

Writing people off like a seventeen-year-old?

When you can identify how old the part of you taking center stage is, think back to what was going on for you in real life back then. Often, you'll find clues as to what's upsetting adult you. For example, if your partner's unilateral decision that you would both attend your nephew's eighth-grade graduation party this weekend has you slamming doors and huffing around like you did at fifteen, it might suggest that adult you is feeling the same lack of self-determination that you did when your parents called the shots. If you can't remember or figure out exactly how old the reactive part is (which, by the by, is very common and doesn't necessarily mean anything about you), try to imagine at roughly what life stage someone might experience the kind of upset you're experiencing: toddler, school age, or teenage.

When you have a sense of how old you're feeling, start by recognizing just how normal your reaction is given the age of your inner child—again, this is a call for understanding and gentleness. A thirty-year-old stomping their foot and screaming isn't ideal, but for a low-resource four-year-old, it makes perfect sense. When you can identify which younger version of you is showing up, it opens the door to much-needed compassion, helping you step out of self-judgment so you can actually shift your behavior and, if needed, make amends to anyone caught in the crossfire. Remember: Staying in judgment keeps you spinning in sympathetic fight-or-flight or detached dorsal shutdown, making it impossible to mobilize, take accountability, or create real change.

Next, try to soothe that inner kiddo the way you wish an adult had comforted you when you were that age (or you sense that a kiddo of that age would want to be comforted). I know for myself that if someone says or implies they know what I'm thinking or feeling more than I do, every twelve- to sixteen-year-old part of me loses it and I shut down. When I start to hear those parts of myself shouting, *You don't know me better than I do!* I know it's time to take space (aka go to the bathroom—the magical space of self-care available in pretty much every setting) and remind her that adult me trusts that she knows herself and, most importantly, to put our focus back on us and our self-love, and not on other people and their projections from their own wounding.

Real self-trust comes from knowing that you will say no to keep your own peace, that you have the skills and capacity to process, understand, and regulate your own emotions. Because you trust that you've got your own back and no longer need other folks to manage your feelings for you, you can ask for support, care, and co-regulation from others when you need and want to. This doesn't mean you're a rock or an island and never seek support or guidance! When you have your own back, you don't need to call every friend and send a thousand pictures before you buy a new pair of jeans or tap-dance feverishly for your dad to approve of you going to culinary school. You know your butt looked damn good, and you're confident that you'll be there to support you even if your dreams of owning a restaurant don't happen quite the way you planned.

It boils down to knowing you can count on you. Knowing you'll be kind to you and won't throw you under the bus. You won't betray or abandon you anymore, no matter how much easier it may feel in the short term. When you have your own back, you know you can count on your own strong sense of emotional intelligence and can navigate emotional challenges with resilience and self-awareness.

While I love theory, your gal is a nurse at the end of the day, so let's talk about a practical way to start rebuilding trust: restorative experiences. In the psychological literature, restorative experiences (alternately called relational or interpersonal restoration) are experiences that you have with other people that restore your faith in humanity after trauma, betrayal, or violation.[7] It's about healing the relationship not just to others, but also to yourself—restoring your belief that you can trust your own judgment and instincts in social connections. In this context, a restorative experience might look like gradually reengaging in relationships where you feel safe, practicing vulnerability in small ways, or finding trustworthy people who respect your boundaries.

When we're just starting our journey to heal Emotional Outsourcing, finding those restorative experiences can be a challenge, so I like to offer my clients a kitten step where we create those self-loving moments to restore faith in ourselves.

To do this, my beautiful blossoming orchid, in a moment where you find yourself overwhelmed with self-criticism after a big ol' failure (or when it just feels like you failed and you didn't even), you're going to follow all those meanie-pants thoughts with a moment of self-compassion. That restorative response might be pausing to put a hand on your heart and say, "I'm learning. I still matter to myself, even if this didn't turn out the way I expected." My client Leia found solace and restoration from sitting in her garden, noticing the new growth around her, and delighting in the reminder that we are all constantly changing.

As you begin to orchestrate restorative experiences for yourself, where you are actively choosing to be kind to you, try to step into the role of that most loving guardian. This is the part of you that offers unconditional love and endless loyalty and kindness and embodies your favorite version of your self. It's the inner voice that offers reassurance, that tells you, *It's okay, you made a mistake, and that doesn't mean you're less worthy—you matter to me, my sweet little tender ravioli.*

CHOOSE KINDER WORDS, PLEASE

My beauty, if being mean to you was going to lead to real, lasting change, it certainly would have worked by now. But it can't and it won't. Trust me, I hear you when you say that it's the only thing that ever has, that you'll be lazy and unmotivated if you don't yell, berate, scold, and shame you. I've told myself that story, and I've heard it a thousand and one times from my clients.

Emotional Outsourcing comes with so much all-or-nothing thinking, and for many of us that meant we were either the super-laudable Good Girl, doing our damnedest to get an A+ and all the extra credit in every area of our lives, or a wicked disappointment, giving up on ourselves before our insufficient attempts prove just how worthless we really are. No matter how you tried to avoid it, both these personas cover up a vicious inner critic. We are so relentlessly mean to ourselves that some of my clients don't have another way of relating to themselves when we first start working together. All they heard growing up—and therefore all they internalized—was criticism or judgment, subtly or overt, and so as adults the only thing they know to believe about themselves is that they are not good enough, that they aren't valuable, and that there's always something they need to do or improve to earn love.

The powers that be aren't exactly helping us either. A super-common example of the way being unkind to ourselves is normalized in our modern, Western culture is the way women, in particular, are taught to feel about our bodies. How many of us know women who fully and unapologetically love themselves and their bodies? It's a rare thing indeed! We are constantly told that to be acceptable and respected we need to look a certain way, have a certain body type, wear certain clothes, style our hair just so. With impossible standards all around us, we rarely see women loving themselves and their bodies modeled for us, and so many of us grew up with parents, especially moms, who are on perma-diets and who talked trash about their looks or bodies all day long—I know I sure did. It's no wonder we think that self-hatred and self-flagellation are the way forward. Not to mention there are entire multi-majillion-dollar industries designed to reinforce the messages that we are flawed and need fixing and very few, if any, industries supporting the idea that self-love is the key to change. No one is making bank off that idea!

The notion that how you talk to yourself is how you think and feel about yourself is supported by plenty of scientific research—all of which suggests that long-term exposure to negative self-talk can have harmful effects on cognitive performance and emotional well-being.[8] These are outcomes I've lived through myself and have witnessed in hundreds of clients. It's clear as can be: In order to shift our underlying stories around self-worth, we have to shift the way we talk to and about ourselves. When you're feeling safer and thus ready to start treating yourself with respect and to affirm your dignity as a person who is whole and worthy even while she is growing, there are three ways you can start shifting your internal culture of meanie-ness:

Talk to an image of your younger self. Did you notice yourself saying something mean? Really laying into yourself for being so stupid and useless? Berating yourself for being a colossal failure and a disappointment? Calling yourself a fat cow or a weak skinny twig? I want you to find a picture of you—ideally as a wee, sweet tender one—and try saying that out loud to her. No, really. Print a picture, hold it in your hand, and say what you just said to yourself to that tiny, beautiful face. Can you do it? Most of us can't—which is the good news. (If you don't have access to a picture of little you, draw one for yourself, using your nondominant hand to evoke the childlike spirit of our kiddo selves.)[9]

One of the great gifts of inner children work is that I'm now more aware of the impact of my self-talk. Anytime I notice my inner critic running amok, I imagine it's speaking to tiny me. It's pretty hard to look my darling, pint-sized self in the eyes and tell her that she's too fat to be lovable, or that she's just so friggin' stupid, or that it's nice and all that she thinks a nap sounds good but she has work to take care of so suck it up. It hits different, my love.

Take out the adjectives. When you notice you're shaming yourself, pause and take out all the adjectives—and especially the swear words. Calling ourselves names and piling on the qualifiers are just ways that we fire that second arrow. You'll be amazed how fast *Why am I such a lazy cussitycusscuss?* loses its sting when it's just *Why am I?*

Ask, "Whose voice is this?" My love, remember, you did not invent these voices of shame and criticism. They are the natural, expected outcome of living in a world that tells you that you aren't worthy unless you're producing, that your feelings and experiences don't matter, that your role is to serve the people around you, full stop. The cruelty and shame that you show yourself are representations of the ways you learned to shut yourself down to survive. By asking "Whose voice is that?" we create space between our emotions and our judgment.

There's no right answer, and maybe even no single answer, but I want you to push past that initial moment of "I don't know . . . mine?" For example, if you look in the mirror and your gaze zeroes in immediately on that "extra" belly you beat yourself up about, pause and ask, *Whose thought is that?* Maybe the disgust that you feel toward your curves is a holdover from a parent's criticism. Or maybe it's shame you picked up from the girls in the locker room in middle school. Maybe it's internalized white Western beauty standards. Perhaps it's the voice of Tyra Banks or Jillian Michaels haunting you from the early 2000s and their respective (extremely popular) TV shows. Maybe it's a combination of the above. Regardless of what answer comes to mind (and even if none surfaces right away), pausing to recognize that maybe, just maybe, you don't want to keep thinking those things about yourself can soften the blow.

I know it can feel challenging, scary, and, yes, cringe to be nice to yourself. And yet! Committing to being a little kinder to yourself every day is pretty nonnegotiable in my humblest opinion. *Ojo*, I said a *little* kinder—not "You have to think the sun and moon and stars of yourself forever and love your thighs and think you fart rainbows all the time starting immediately," 'cause that's some BS. It's all about those kitten steps: one moment where you choose compassion or a gentle word over self-recrimination. One "of course I did" instead of throwing yourself under every available bus. It all adds up. Doing your level best to pause, breathe, and choose kindness (or even just not cruelty), especially when it's hard, is how you teach yourself that you are worthy of love and care in your own eyes—starting by showing you you're not totally worthless, no matter what those gremlins in your head may be saying.

Kitten Step: Pick Your Own Pet Name

You've probably noticed, my delectable pickled pepper, that I have been using a *lot* of pet names in this book. Like, *a lot* a lot. Well, that's not just a personality quirk—it's by design (and also because I'm Argentine and we love a good nickname, *petisa linda*!). You see, one of the easiest ways to bring in kinder self-talk is to call yourself sweet little names on the regular (#BecauseScience). It's something I've been doing for myself over the years with beautiful results, and once my clients adjust to the initial strangeness or clash with some Waspier ways of relating, they love doing it for themselves too—and every listener of my podcast, *Feminist Wellness*, knows that I think they are a perfect little tender ravioli—and you are too!

It feels really good to be kind to me and say, "Oh, you sweet, silly little bunny! Look at you making a real goose-up of it!" in a little singsong voice when I eff up versus being my own perpetrator. It makes the experience of failure so much more gentle, which helps keep my nervous system in ventral vagal, thus holding space for me to actually learn, take responsibility, and grow—not just spin in meanness. *Science!**

Depending on your own journey through Emotional Outsourcing, you may find it mildly to moderately or even wicked-hella very, very challenging to embrace acts of kindness, tenderness, and pet names for so many reasons. For real, growing up in Waspy homes with no emotions can do it! Also, when we grow up in emotionally immature homes, we may smartly learn to avoid vulnerability to protect our tender hearts, leading us to perceive expressions of care as openings to our emotional fragility, so of course we bat these gestures away, using the survival skill of denying kindness as a way to guard against exposing our innermost selves and human vulnerability. Makes total sense—of course you did. Many of us also learned to prioritize self-reliance and self-sufficiency to avoid leaning on unreliable folks, which of course makes us uncomfortable with expressions of care that may imply putting our eggs in other people's baskets when that maybe didn't work out so well in the past. And for sure it's often very cultural to not be very warm or cuddly, even in our word choices, and we always want to honor that lineage of stiff-upper-lippedness while inviting you to give kind self-talk the ol' college try.

I'll invite you to try this on by picking a pet name for yourself. It can be silly, it can be traditional, it can be a favorite from childhood or a book or movie—whatever makes you feel held and cared for in a way that doesn't make you want to run screaming from the whole project. Then, in the next few hours, see if you can work it into a moment of self-talk. It doesn't have to be anything big: a quick "All right, tiger, it's time for some lunch" or "*Reina mía*, you really need to get a move on or you're going to be late again this morning" can be enough to begin to soften your attitude

* Okay, so, this isn't really based in science per se, like I don't have a white paper or study to point to, it's based in my experience of life, but it's really fun to declare Science! So… Science!

toward yourself and can help you recognize your own dignity, buried under all that self-doubt and meanie-ness. As your capacity to sit with self-kindness grows, see if your moments of gentle, loving self-talk can grow too, you perfect little olive leaf!

YOU'RE THE CAKE!

Everything we've been talking about in this chapter brings us around to my most beloved *metáfora*: Be the Cake. I believe that each of us is like a scrumptious many-layer cake: We are complete entities—delicious, whole, and sufficient in ourselves. For sure we can add frosting (other people's affirmation, validations, etc.) because who doesn't love a little extra chocolate buttercream? The key thing is wanting it without feeling graspy or telling the story that we have to contort or chameleon ourselves for it because we *need* it. Reveling in our cakeness is the goal—to believe that you are whole, worthy of all good things, scrumptious and desirable exactly as you are. The icing is just the icing—something that we are strong enough in our self-story to welcome without believing we aren't complete without it.

When we live from our Emotional Outsourcing habits, we become obsessed with how the cake of self looks—especially how it looks to others. We fret over the buttercream roses, the placement of the sprinkles, whether the frosting is smooth enough. We get so fixated on the outside—on making sure we appear "good enough" in other people's eyes—that we forget to actually *be someone*—to actually be our Self in this life. It's like spending all our energy icing an empty cake pan instead of baking something real. To put it plainly, my darling: Codependent, perfectionist, and people-pleasing habits keep us trapped in a loop of seeking external validation, worrying about how we're perceived rather than anchoring into who we truly are.

Self-compassion, self-trust, and positive self-regard—shaped by the way we talk to ourselves—are the key ingredients of our cake. When those are in place, we can live our lives knowing that we are the main event. When you're the cake, you know you're incredible just as you are. You welcome others into your life not because you need their approval to feel worthy, but because you know you're better together. From this place of embodied cakeness, you can fully enjoy the sweetness of affirmation—"Wow! You crushed that presentation today!" or "Thank you for dinner, it was delicious!" or "Your hair looks amazing!"—without needing it to prove your worth. The love and support of those around you will always add beauty and joy to life, but as the cake, your pride, confidence, and self-respect aren't up for debate. They are yours, baked right into who you are.

Take my client Clara, for example. She managed an international team for a large tech company, and for as long as she could remember, she slept with her phone under her pillow, ringer on. If she got an email, she'd rub the sleep from her bleary eyes and reply instantly—even at 4 a.m. Burnout was her baseline, and she teetered on the edge of full-blown physical collapse but also reported feeling "fine, thanks." Her irritable bowel syndrome was out of control, and she'd gotten walking pneumonia twice that year already (which, of course, she'd worked straight through). Her doctors warned her that if she didn't get a handle on her sleep and stress, she'd be looking at serious, long-term health impacts.

In coaching, we worked on all of this—but at its core, we were working on how she saw herself. Clara had spent years believing that her worth was tied to her responsiveness, to being needed, to proving—again and again—that she was indispensable. I introduced her to the idea that she wasn't just the decorator fussing over the buttercream, anxiously trying to make everything perfect for everyone else. She was the cake. Her worth wasn't in how well she performed for others—it was already baked in.

One morning, after waking to a not-at-all-urgent update from an engineer based in the Netherlands, she sat at the edge of her bed, holding her phone, and realized she couldn't remember the last time she had slept through the night. Exhausted, she felt a pang of anger and then a flash of clarity. A quiet, unfamiliar question surfaced: *What if I mattered?* she wondered. *What if **my** well-being mattered just as much as my team's well-being? What if I, and not my team, were the cake? What if it's not a problem that they don't hear from me until morning?* The realization hit her like a tidal wave, and she knew something had to change. Clara decided to start small: She began turning her phone on silent mode at 10 p.m. and placing it in the living room instead of under her pillow. The first night, she barely slept, anxious about the potential chaos she might find in her inbox the next morning. But to her surprise, the world didn't fall apart. Over the next few weeks, she stuck to her boundaries and discovered that her team managed just fine without her midnight responses. Gradually, Clara began to prioritize her sleep and set clearer limits, making herself—and her well-being—the foundation of her workday. And most importantly, she let herself be the main event in her own life.

Not just a boon to our sense of self, adopting the "Be the Cake" mind-set fosters healthier interpersonal relationships, encouraging us to engage in relationships not out of perceived necessity or a sense of incompleteness, but from a place of wholeness and self-assurance. This shift in perspective leads to more balanced and fulfilling interactions, where relationships enhance life rather than define it.

To practice being the cake (drum roll, please...), we focus on developing self-awareness and self-compassion. Yup, that's right: We go right back to the top of the chapter and keep on kitten-stepping our way through "of course I did," pet names, and words of kindness. We continue to cultivate our Watcher and evidence to our inner kiddos through consistent repetition that we are someone we can count on—because we are the cake!

Examples of Being the Cake (to Inspire You!)

- Saying "No, that doesn't work for me" without over-explaining or apologizing.
- Taking yourself out to dinner at your favorite spot—just because you *want* to.
- Deleting the unsent text asking if they're mad at you and choosing to trust the relationship instead.
- Feeling the pull to overfunction and choosing to sit in the discomfort *without fixing.*
- Letting yourself rest *before* you burn out—not waiting until exhaustion forces you.
- Celebrating your own win—even if no one else notices.
- Holding a boundary, even when someone is disappointed, and reminding yourself: *Their feelings are theirs to manage.*
- Buying yourself flowers instead of waiting for someone else to think of it.
- Walking away from a conversation that disrespects your worth, even if you used to stay and justify.
- Looking in the mirror, seeing your own softness and strength, and thinking: *I am enough, exactly as I am.*
- And of course, complimenting your own gorgeous mane: You look stunning, darling!

JOURNAL PROMPTS
WHAT'S YOUR FLAVOR OF CAKE?

Being the cake takes time and persistence. When we're not used to being the center of gravity in our own lives, it can feel unfamiliar—even challenging—to affirm our worth and recognize all the incredible ways we already show up. All the beautiful, unique pieces that make up our authentic self. All the beautiful, unique pieces that comprise our authentic self. As you work to compassionately have your own back, I invite you to spend some extra time exploring what makes you you, and what might be holding you back from knowing just how valuable, lovable, and special you are.

1. **What are the ingredients that make up my sense of self?**
   Take time to list the qualities, values, and strengths that you know are part of who you are, independent of others' opinions. The things you like about you or find okay-enough.

2. **How do self-compassion, self-trust, and positive self-regard show up in my life right now?**
   What could life look like if you lived it with more of these self-loving/kinder habits?

3. **Where in my life am I chasing the icing more than appreciating the cake?**
   Reflect on the moments when you've sought external validation or approval over your own self-regard or opinion. What emotions, beliefs, or stories drove you to focus on what others think instead of recognizing your own worth? Where did you learn to do that?

   ....

   ....

   ....

4. **How would I feel if the icing of others' praise or validation wasn't available?**
   Consider a situation where you're looking for praise or approval. Now imagine that you don't get it. What would that stir up in you? Where do you feel the discomfort of not receiving external affirmation, and how could you soothe that from within?

   ....

   ....

   ....

5. **What is one recent moment when I was the cake—when I acted from a place of knowing I was complete and whole?**
   Write about a time when you made a choice that came from your self-worth. How did it feel to move from that place of wholeness? How did others react, and how did it shape your experience? If you can't think of one that really happened, dream one up!

   ....

   ....

   ....

6. **When do I notice myself decorating the empty cake pan instead of baking the cake?**
   Are there moments in your life where you're focusing on outward appearances or perfectionism rather than nourishing your deeper sense of self? How can you shift from worrying about appearances to strengthening your internal core?

   ....

   ....

   ....

7. **What does my cake need right now to be even more nourishing and satisfying?**
   Think of your emotional, mental, and physical needs. How can you add more self-compassion, self-trust, or positive self-regard to your daily life to nourish yourself as you are, without relying on external validation?

   ....

   ....

   ....

8. **How can I celebrate being the cake, just as I am?**
   Brainstorm small ways to acknowledge your accomplishments, your strengths, and the beauty of who you are, even if no one else is watching. What would it look like to throw a party for your inner cake without needing anyone else to bring the frosting?

   ....

   ....

   ....

9. **How do I show up in relationships when I believe I'm the cake?**
   Reflect on your relationships from the perspective that you are already whole. How does this shift your behaviors, thoughts, and feelings in connection with others? How might your relationships feel lighter and more fulfilling from this place?

   ....

   ....

   ....

10. **What stories do I tell myself about needing the icing?**
    Write about the narratives you've internalized about why you need others' validation or approval. How true do they feel, and where did these stories come from? How might they change if you embraced your cakeness more fully?

    ....

    ....

    ....

11. **How can I support myself in being the cake when old patterns of Emotional Outsourcing show up?**
    What are some tools or strategies you can use to gently remind yourself of your wholeness when you start to notice people-pleasing, perfectionism, or codependency habits creeping in?

    ....

    ....

    ....

Chapter 6

Somatics 101

Whenever I give a lecture on somatics, I start by asking my audience to raise their hand if they identify with "living from the neck up." Without fail, hands shoot up like I just asked who wanted an all-expenses-paid work-free vacation to the beach of their choice, and I'm hardly surprised. When we grow up the way we did, which trains us to believe that what's happening outside of us is more important than what's happening inside of us, it's little wonder that so many of us folks struggling with Emotional Outsourcing have disconnected from our bodies. At the common advice to "listen to your body," we scoff, "I don't even speak the same language as this weird skin suit. What has it done for me lately?" Having learned that a real, embodied awareness of our physical needs or feelings is risky, our nervous system turns off the proverbial tap, encouraging us to brain our way through since body is apparently unreliable or unsafe.

Remember back in chapter 3 when we learned about functional freeze? Caught between the need to source safety through doing and the overwhelming fear that we are failing and may never do enough to merit care, love, and connection from those around us, our nervous system stalls out in this mixed state that's a bit sympathetic, a bit dorsal, and keeps us at arm's length from being embodied in our own reality.

I want to emphasize again that there is absolutely nothing wrong with your body or your nervous system if you are living in functional freeze or any other state. When you're constantly getting pushed (or shoved) outside your window of capacity, *of course* your nervous system will do whatever it can to keep you safe and alive, 'cause that's its job.

It's also a lousy way to live. Disconnecting from our bodies shuts us down to our own needs, wants, desires, emotions, and truths. You don't know whether you're thirsty or hungry, let alone whether you can trust yourself to choose the right career, home, romantic partner, outfit, or belief system for you.

My dazzling, brave blueberry, I know you want to know yourself again—the *real* you who's been pushed down all these years. What I need to say loud and clear is that the work to come home to yourself, to step out of the codependent, perfectionist, and people-pleasing habits that limit your capacity for reciprocal, nourishing relationships, doesn't just happen in your head. You can think all the "right" thoughts and notice your patterns 'til the cows come home. But the healing won't stick—and in some cases just plain can't happen—without showing your nervous system that you're actually safe and okay.* We need to get back in touch

---

* And I need to name this: *Not everyone has the privilege of feeling safe in their own body.* When systems of oppression—white supremacy, patriarchy, fatphobia, ableism, transphobia—mark some bodies as more worthy of safety than others, nervous system healing can't be separated from the reality of living in those systems. If your body has never been treated as safe, seen, or valued, of course safety doesn't just "land" because you practice regulation. Of course vigilance, hyperawareness, and bracing feel like second nature. This work doesn't ask you to gaslight yourself into believing you're safe when you're not—but to start carving out moments, however small, where safety can be *cultivated*, where your body can *experience* just a little more ease, even within a world that makes it hard.

with our bodies, and to do that, we gotta speak its language: the language of somatics.

WHAT IS SOMATICS AGAIN?

The term "somatic" comes from the Greek word *soma*, meaning "the living body" or "the body in its wholeness." Somatic practices encompass a variety of tools that help us experience our bodies, minds, and spirits as an integrated, interconnected system.[1] But let's be clear: *Indigenous cultures across the globe have always known this.* Long before the West coined the term "somatics," embodied wisdom was central to Indigenous traditions—through dance, ritual movement, song, storytelling, breathwork, and healing practices that honored the body's innate intelligence.[2] Thanks to Eurocentric paradigms (looking at you, Descartes![*]), the West compartmentalized mind and body, repressing or erasing these long-standing traditions in favor of the belief that humans are—and should be—creatures of the mind alone.

But, turtledove, that's not how humans work. If you've ever felt butterflies in your stomach before a big presentation, watched weeks of stress become an unwelcome pimple right on your chin, or felt the physical heaviness of grief weigh you down, you already know that your emotions can and do manifest physically. Science and basic anatomy evidence that there is a bidirectional relationship between mind and body, where the vagus nerve is the superhighway between the two.[3] Translation? Your thoughts, feelings, and memories can show up as physical experiences, and vice versa—what's happening in your body influences how you think, feel, and act in each moment.

---

* René Descartes of "I think, therefore I am" fame developed the philosophy that came to define the West's belief in an immutable mind-body split (which we call Cartesian dualism).

Nobody exemplified this better than my client María Soledad, who grew up with a doctor mom and a stressed-out teacher dad, neither one of whom regularly attuned to her or her siblings. Sol developed irritable bowel syndrome as a young teen, and her mom, who had lost her own mother early, was so freaked out by the possibility of her baby being sick that she shut down any conversation around Sol's health without realizing what she was doing. Fast-forward forty years, and the moment María Soledad feels even a twinge in her stomach, panic sets in—intensifying her symptoms, which then fuel more panic, until she's caught in a full-blown flare-up *and* a side of ye olde panic attack, as her body and mind keep locking each other in a feedback loop.

Somatic practices as we understand them today all trade on this fundamental belief in the mind-body connection. Instead of working exclusively from the top down (i.e., privileging the mind), somatic modalities allow us to work from the bottom up and engage our bodies to access, accompany, and ultimately heal chronic nervous system dysregulation. We do this because true healing isn't just about understanding our pain—it's about *repatterning* the body's response to it, creating new pathways for safety, connection, and resilience. The result? A life where we're no longer ruled by old survival strategies, where we can move through the world with more ease, self-trust, and the capacity for deep, reciprocal relationships—*and find ourselves snapping at customer service or our kids way less often.*

RESOURCING: HAVING YOUR NERVOUS SYSTEM'S BACK

Growing up in Emotional Outsourcing, we learn to hide away our true needs and experiences—whether that's acknowledging that you're tired or need to pee, knowing what you want for dinner, or noticing how hurtful and alienating a friend's criticism really is. We learned early and often to stuff down emotions that were unwelcome or unpopular with our caregivers. We learned to ignore our biological impulses, like ignoring a need to use the bathroom at every rest stop on a long road trip to not be "annoying" to Dad and thus risk exclusion or ridicule. You were sure to be praised by your caregivers when you didn't cry, no matter how upset you were about the ice cream cone gone belly-up on the sidewalk, so you held it in—sucked it up, buttercup—and did the same when your husband never lifted a finger or your partner wasn't supportive of your dreams. And who has time to be hungry in the face of a modern workplace culture where, if you wanted to be taken seriously and get that promotion, you'd better learn to inhale half a protein bar while multitasking between meetings.

Overlooking our body's signals, or biological impulses, is a form of learned self-neglect and self-abandonment—precisely the comfortable discomfort that our nervous system learned would keep us safe as kiddos. So often our own emotions seem too overwhelming after a lifetime of avoiding them (and never learning how to feel them in the first place). By the time we're adults, we're so habituated to living outside our window of capacity (stranded in functional freeze) that we can no longer connect inward. Deaf to our own needs and desires, we're left to rely on the opinions and experiences of others to tell us if we're safe, if we matter, and if we're welcome—we rely on the icing, forgetting we're the cake, leaving our nervous system dangling in the proverbial wind.

My love, we cannot truly shake our Emotional Outsourcing survival skills until we learn to be present *in* and *with* our bodies—and to craft new skills that aren't just about survival, but about *presence, choice, and true embodiment.* Skills that let us respond instead of react, that anchor us in our own experience instead of outsourcing our worth, that make space for connection without self-abandonment. And that's why somatic practices are so wicked vital to learn. Somatics are how we work with our bodies to source safety and regain our capacity to move through the polyvagal ladder without getting stuck. By learning tools to regulate ourselves on purpose, with compassion and kindness, we invite our nervous system to see that it's safe to thaw that functional freeze. The more time we spend in regulation, the more our window of capacity can relax and widen, creating a cycle where we don't get quite so dysregulated quite so often and are able to put smart boundaries up or otherwise protect ourselves when the environment *actually* isn't safe. Through this process we gain choicefulness, which is the greatest gift of this work.

While I'm thrilled there is more somatics education in the world, I'm troubled by the context-less nervous system "hacks" like heel drops and humming "voo" that have taken over many of our social media feeds. They're sexy, seemingly miraculous interventions to "calm" your nervous system as though that were a panacea for all that ails. Many of these tools are genuinely effective for nervous system regulation, and as a nurse practitioner and somatic experiencing practitioner, I'm all for anything that's science-based and practical. The trouble is that many are offered up as Band-Aids. It's like taking a handful of Tums: It might stem the pain of that chronic heartburn temporarily, but it's not getting to the root of why you have heartburn to begin with. Similarly, you can hold ice cubes when you're stressing as many times as you need to, but it's not going to have a sustained impact on your window of capacity. For that we're going to have to resource our nervous systems and also do the deep social justice work that makes for a more kind, just, and equitable world for all of us. "No justice, no peace" applies to our nervous systems too.

Resourcing is the intentional practice of giving our nervous system the experiences, tools, and support it needs to regulate—not by eliminating dysregulation, but by increasing our capacity to navigate it. Regulation isn't about staying calm at all times; it's about staying present with ourselves when dysregulation happens, rather than defaulting to habitual coping strategies and self-abandoning. It's about cultivating a sense of internal safety, even in the face of activation.[4] Coping strategies, by contrast, numb us to and disconnect us from that activation. They're the buffering, overfunctioning, and ruminating we explored in chapter 4 (among other habits)—the adaptive ways we learned to function *despite* nervous system dysregulation. Because let's be real: Staying in a heightened state of activation forever isn't an option. It's overwhelming, exhausting, and unsustainable.

Meanwhile, regulating resources do something entirely different. Instead of simply masking dysregulation, they help us move through it, allowing stored activation to discharge from our system. Regulating resources create a felt sense of safety and connection in the body, whether through internal practices like breath awareness, somatic grounding, or mindful attention, or external supports like trusted relationships, soothing environments, or familiar rituals—a warm bath, a favorite scent, the well-worn pages of a beloved book.

At its core, resourcing is about reminding the nervous system: *You are not in danger in this moment.* It's what allows us to shift out of survival mode and into a state where we can rest, digest, connect, and *truly live.*[5]

Our nervous system is constantly responding to internal and external stimuli. When we resource, we give it the chance to settle and recalibrate, helping to prevent long-term dysregulation that can feed into chronic stress, anxiety, or burnout. Resourcing helps to expand our window of capacity—the zone within which we can experience emotions, stressors, and challenges without becoming overwhelmed. With a wider window, we can navigate life's ups and downs without spiraling into fight or flight (sympathetic activation) or shutdown (dorsal vagal collapse).

In the context of Emotional Outsourcing, resourcing the nervous system is vital because when we are dysregulated, we are far more likely to rely on external validation, approval, or soothing to feel okay—we have less access to make mindful, intentional choices for our lives because we start running on default habits. A well-resourced nervous system is more adaptable. It's better equipped to handle the emotional, mental, and physical challenges that come our way, and it helps us return to a regulated state faster after we've been triggered.[6] When we are resourced and regulated, we are more capable of engaging in meaningful, authentic connection with others.

So, nerd that I am, in the next few pages I'm going to help you fill your toolbox with five evidence-based practices I trust will shore up your window of capacity and teach your nervous system that you've got its back: orienting, grounding, body scan, soothing recall, and glimmers. This is by no means an exhaustive list (I teach more than two dozen to my clients in my six-month program, Anchored, and in my somatic workshops and seminars), but dollars to doughnuts these five will give you the foundation you need to allow your body to begin to rebuild its trust that regulation is safe and possible (something that years of Emotional Outsourcing have likely eroded).

You can—and should!—call on these tools in moments of dysregulation, and they'll have the most impact if you also practice them during moments of relative ease and calm, when you're solidly in ventral vagal. Consistency and repetition will gift your nervous system the attunement and reassurance that it needs to believe that adult you has got this. The more you can count on yourself and trust that you're capable of managing your emotional states independently, the less reliant you will be on those codependent, perfectionist, and people-pleasing scripts and habits to attempt to source safety.

A Reminder about Safety

Somatic work is challenging, my love. We have stored years of repressed fear, anguish, loneliness, pain, stress, and distress in our nervous systems, and I won't pretend that it isn't overwhelming to start acknowledging and getting in touch with those emotions. This is even more true for folks who are living with histories of trauma, such as sexual assault or domestic violence, eating disorders, or living in a marginalized/othered body. With this in mind, I want you to remember those kitten steps, *mi amor.* Go slowly. If something feels like too much, leave it. *Basta.* That's enough in that moment. Don't perfectionist-all-or-nothing your way through these exercises because you're "supposed to," to heal. No, thank you! That's actually going to create the opposite effect—you trust yourself less instead of more. So just notice the emotion or sensation that's coming up, then back off and try an Anchor Scan, which you'll learn in a jiff. Strong-arming your nervous system into distress does nothing to teach your nervous system that you've got its back.

You don't need to go this alone, my love. Support from a therapist, well-trained coach, or counselor can be so helpful. If at any point you are worried that you may self-harm or have suicidal thoughts, call 988 or emergency support in your area. You are loved.

ORIENTING

One of the best ways to invite our nervous systems into regulation is to orient ourselves in the present, and this is a vital thing to do before, and sometimes during and after, doing one of these practices. Orienting the nervous system is what makes these practices less like Band-Aids and more likely to actually help shift things for you. When our nervous systems are triggered—sending us further into either sympathetic activation or dorsal shutdown—we lose touch with the immediacy of our surroundings and precisely when and where we are. Our body, screaming "Danger!" believes that it's back in the situation where we first learned that stimulus was dangerous and acts accordingly. In other words, you feel about six years old and scared (even though the grown-ups said it was stupid and that you needed to be a big girl), or fourteen years old and in a moving truck, driving away from the only home you've ever known because your parents sold it in the divorce, and you don't have access to your adult skills and nervous system—inner children are driving the Trigger Truck.

My client Taylor knew this time-travel feeling well: Every night without fail, cornered in the whirlwind of her children's demands and her husband's underfunctioning indifference, she jumped into the Fixer role, overfunctioning like a champ. At a loss, she bribed the kids to not be monsters with promises of extra *Bluey* episodes and talked incessantly to attempt to keep her husband engaged. Physically she was there at the family table monitoring the distance between the chicken nuggets and the ketchup, ready to swoop in at any moment to avoid a Chernobyl-level toddler meltdown should the dread red touch the pristine tenders, while emotionally, she was back at her own childhood dinner table, telling jokes to get the attention of her taciturn father and kicking her younger sibling under the table when they got too rowdy so Mom wouldn't yell or melt down herself.

In those moments when our nervous system jolts us into the past, orienting is a quick and simple tool to remind it that we are adults,[7] not little kiddos in danger, and that we aren't in the same situation where we learned what unsafe felt like—we have skills and tools now. We orient our nervous system the same way you'd orient someone to your home if they were visiting: "This is the kitchen, this is the guest room, the bathroom is down the hall, and here is my beloved collection of snow globes from around the world." We pointedly notice our environment. By grounding ourselves in the details of where we are right now in the present moment, especially through our senses and not just our minds, we can encourage our body to neurocept safety and help our nervous system find its way back into regulation.

You may have heard of the 5-4-3-2-1 technique, where you identify five things that you can see, four you can touch, three you can hear, two you can smell, and one you can taste as a way to engage your senses fully in your surroundings and help bring your logical mind back online.[8] Other forms look like focusing on a nearby object, exploring details like color, texture, and weight in your clothes or the items on your desk, or speaking facts like your name, the date, and your location out loud (or in your mind depending on where you are), to remind yourself that you are here and present in the moment.

My personal favorite, the Anchor Scan, pulls double duty by engaging your mind (prefrontal cortex) *and* your body to bring yourself back into the present. Here's how it goes:

- Start by looking all the way over your left shoulder, and then—slowly, slowly, slowly—swivel your head so that you're looking over your right shoulder (or vice versa). As you do, notice and name (out loud if it's safe to do so) what you're seeing in your environment: window, plant, pens, computer, crystal, coffee, cat, and so on.
- On the second pass (moving your head from right back to left), choose a shape or color and focus on all the items you see that match. For example, if you pick the color yellow, maybe you notice the citrine gemstone, a highlighter, a yellow leaf on a plant, the warm sunshine in the window. Or maybe you choose "circle" and bring your attention to the way your cat is curled up tight, a coffee mug, the pot holding your pens, and a flower.
- On your third pass (again, and *ever so slowly*, swiveling your head from left to right), name one thing you can hear, smell, or taste: your cat's purr, coffee.
- Continue moving your head and naming patterns in your environment until you can take a full, complete breath, perhaps sigh or otherwise notice a state change—your body coming back toward ventral vagal.

What's so effective about the Anchor Scan is its one-two punch: Noticing patterns gives your mind something rote and predictable to do, which helps bring your prefrontal cortex back online,[9] while swiveling your head tells your nervous system that you don't have to be locked down, eyes front for danger,[10] and that it's okay to relax into greater felt safety.[11] Again, practice it when you don't *need* it so it's your second nature go-to when you do.

GROUNDING

Grounding is orienting's favorite cousin.[12] Where orienting brings us back to the present through our sensory connection to the world outside of ourselves, grounding connects us to our environment and the earth through our bodies and is so helpful when we're feeling emotionally or physically overwhelmed. Grounding techniques aim to bring attention back into the body and create a sense of safety and stability by engaging the senses—think about feeling your feet on the floor, the texture of an object in your hands, or the rhythm of your breath as it moves through you. If orienting says, "I'm here, and my environment is safe," grounding says, "I'm here, and I am safe within myself."

When we're stuck in functional freeze, we've disconnected from our Self, so much so that my clients often describe a sensation of floating through the world instead of moving through it with intention. Whether you're revved up and running too fast to feel or are so detached from your own wants, needs, mind, and body that you don't quite feel tethered to the world around you, your nervous system needs to feel something sturdy underneath you to feel safe.

Grounding is about helping your nervous system know that it's safe and supported—in this case quite literally. The goal of grounding is to feel solidness underneath you and to draw stability from the earth, Pachamama, or whatever you call her, beneath your feet, from the chair you're sitting on, the subway car you're riding in, or even the sturdiness of your own body. You don't have to balance your nervous system's reactions on the unpredictable ground of others' opinions, kitten. When we learn to ground and access self-support, we can stand confidently in our own bodies and the surety of the ground beneath our feet, even when it's many stories below our apartment.

This practice can be especially helpful when you need to regain composure in the moment or before doing a scary thing. If you notice that your thoughts are racing, you feel on edge after an activating or triggering event, or you feel disconnected or dissociated from your body or reality, try grounding yourself in the earth and getting embodied (present in your body) through one or more of the following practices:

- **Progressive muscle relaxation:** This technique helps release physical tension by consciously tightening and relaxing muscles. Find a quiet place to sit or lie down. Starting with your toes, curl them tightly for a count of 5, then release. Move up to your feet, legs, stomach, hands, arms, and shoulders, tensing each muscle group for a count of 5, and then relaxing. After tensing and relaxing each part of your body, take a deep breath and notice how much more relaxed your muscles feel.
- **Movement:** Engage in simple movements like stretching, walking, or gently swaying side to side (bonus points if you can get outside and connect with natural elements like grass, trees, or the sky while you move).
- **Run water over your hands:** Start by running cool water over your open palms. Focus on how the temperature feels on each part of your hand, from your wrist to your nails. Switch to warm water and focus on how the sensation on your hands changes.

While any of these can be a helpful quick fix, grounding techniques are most helpful when practiced regularly, not just in moments of distress. Regular practice helps build resilience and a stronger connection to the present, making it easier to stay in our window of capacity and bodily dignity, which slowly expands the more we orient and ground. So simple! So effective!

Kitten Step: *Long* Exhale

It takes practice to feel the support of your body and the world around you. One simple, super-science-supported way to begin is by grounding in your breath. By controlling the cadence of our breathing we can change the signals our nervous system receives, reduce stress hormone production, and shift ourselves back toward regulation.[13] There are tons of breathwork strategies out there, and focusing on a long, *s-l-o-w* exhale, especially while orienting, is my favorite way to calm ourselves. So, as a kitten step, here's what I'd like you to try right now in this moment:

- Inhale for 4 counts.
- Exhale for 8 counts.
- Repeat 2 more times for a total of 3 breaths.
- Notice how you feel before and after.

If you can't breathe in for 4 or out for 8, no worries, my sweet! All bodies are different, and chronic dysregulation can really do a number on your diaphragm (the muscle that controls your inhales and exhales).[14] What's most important is that long, slow exhale, so try your best to breathe out for double the count you breathe in. For example, if you inhale for 3, exhale for 6.

BODY SCAN

When we live from a habit of Emotional Outsourcing, we tend to focus all our attention outward: *What are they feeling? What do they think about me? Are they hungry? I should put my work down and go make them some food. They're doing that thing they do when their shoulder hurts—should I make an appointment for PT?* We focus our attention outside our self so often and so habitually that many of us actually forget to tune in to our own bodies. (Speaking of which, darling succulent, when was the last time you had a sip of water? How about a snack? Where are your shoulders right now? Are they below your ears? Let's roll those out real quick.)

Part of teaching our nervous system that it is safe with adult us is showing our body that we can listen to and correctly interpret its signals most of the time. As an added bonus, when we evidence that we are attuned to our own needs and emotions, our bodies don't have to scream so loudly for our attention in the form of gut issues, sleep issues, and the myriad consequences of hormonal imbalance, so that's fun!

Also called *somatic attunement*, body scans are a mindfulness technique that leverages purposeful, focused attention to the sensations within our bodies—and, no, I didn't make this up; it's a practice as old as time.[15] Over the long term, this exercise can help us link emotions, bodily sensation, and our habitual reactions to life, giving us more insight and more influence in our nervous system's reactions.

Before we explore the practice, I want to say that I recommend doing a body scan once a day at first to build awareness of and presence in your body . . . *with one caveat*. For those of us with a trauma history, body scans are often a mixed bag. On the one hand, somatic attunement can facilitate reconnection with our bodies. Cultivating nonjudgment and curiosity about our bodies can help us approach the trauma they've been holding for us with compassion, rather than avoidance or fear, fostering our capacity to sit with those feelings. On the other *very, very important* hand: Being present in your body can be existentially challenging for folks with trauma histories. Particularly when the body was the site of that trauma, as it is for survivors of rape, sexual assault, physical or emotional abuse, and also frequently for folks existing in marginalized bodies, your body may be holding reservoirs of pain that are too much to access right now or on your own. The point of resourcing your nervous system is to offer it safety; if being in your body isn't a safe choice for you today, don't do it.

Here's how the body scan works: In a safe, comfortable space, we're going to slowly move our attention through the body, noticing what's happening in each part, without any pressure to change what we find. If at any point your mind wanders off or feels too overwhelmed, no biggie. Invite yourself back to your breath and continue with the scan, extending gentle, loving curiosity.

- Start by orienting your nervous system to your surroundings, using an Anchor Scan if you'd like, which we do before any and all somatic practices in my world.
- Then find a comfortable position. You can sit with your feet on the ground, lie down, or even do this walking—whatever feels good to you. If it feels safe to do so, gently close your beautiful eyes or simply soften your gaze. Take a deep breath in, followed by a long, slow exhale.
- When you're ready, move your attention to the soles of your feet. Feel them there with you and notice if they feel warm or cold, tense or relaxed. Note any numbness, disconnection, tingling, or tightness. Pause for the length of at least 2 breaths as you give your full attention to the physical sensations you feel in your feet.
- Slowly, slowly, move your attention up to your ankles, and ask the same questions—are they warm or cold?

Tense or relaxed? Again, notice if there's any numbness, disconnection, tingling, or tightness, any other sensation.
- Continue to gently shift your attention up your body, moving through your calves, shins, knees, thighs, hips, stomach, low back, chest, shoulders, arms, neck, and head, each time pausing to note the physical sensations that are present. Warm or cold? Tense or relaxed? Where do you feel numbness, disconnection, tingling, or tightness?
- If it feels safe, allow yourself to soften. Release your brow, your jaw, your abdomen, your calves.
- To finish, take one deep, full-body breath, from the crown of your head to the tips of your toes, with that long, slow exhale we practiced. Flutter open your eyes and, if you'd like, complete an Anchor Scan (page 183) to come back to presence.

If it feels foreign, strange, or uncomfortable, that's okay. It can be pretty weird the first couple of times for sure. There's no wrong way to do a body scan, and nothing to achieve here. You don't need to feel anything profound or life-changing or to stay focused and not have thoughts (brains are gonna brain, after all). The magic is just in the noticing. Body scans are a practice, and like any practice, the more you do it, the more familiar (and less weird feeling) it becomes. You're building a relationship with your body and with yourself, and that is always a worthy pursuit.

It's normal if you feel absolutely nothing; it's also completely normal if a *lot* starts coming up during a body scan. It's not uncommon for me to notice folks crying, shaking, even full-blown sobbing when I coach body scans in my somatic seminars and with my clients. I know for myself how surprising and (at first) frightening it can be to start bawling outta nowhere: I remember doing a guided meditation at a yoga class, chilling and checking in on how my hips were feeling and *bam!* sobbing. If that's you, my love,

I promise there is nothing wrong. It's just your body and nervous system moving some of those feelings it's been holding on to for you all these years. Let it out, orient, drop the need to understand it and consider just being with it, and then thank yourself for taking the time to check in and to listen.

Kitten Step: Find Your Feet

Sheila, like a lot of my clients, had a tough time with body scans initially. Every time she'd sit down to notice her body, her nervous system resisted *hard*, offering lots of distraction and ever-longer lists of Urgent Things to Do in the Other Room, and if she didn't stop focusing inward she would spiral fast toward anxiety and even panic.

Distractions are natural when we're not used to being present in our bodies. Most of the time, we can simply breathe through them—gently refocusing the mind and gradually building our capacity to stay with what is. We honor that our nervous systems learned that it was best for our survival if we pay very little to no attention to the body behind the curtain. That said, breathing through it is one thing, and forcing yourself too far beyond your window of capacity is another altogether. Pushing the body (versus gently encouraging yourself) only entrenches your nervous system's belief that listening to self is too overwhelming and therefore marks self-awareness as capital-*U* unsafe. In other words: Doing a body scan won't do you any good if it causes big anxiety or a panic attack.

If you're in the same boat as Sheila, I recommend that you start with the kitten step of just noticing your feet. See if you can feel them pressing down on the floor, or how they feel in your socks. Over time, paying attention to the sensation in your feet won't feel as threatening to your nervous system, and your body may start to allow you to notice other parts of your body too.

SOOTHING RECALL

Here's something magical about our beautifully intelligent bodies: They don't actually need to be physically present with a calming person or energy to feel calmed. When we vividly imagine calming scenes or experiences, people or animals, the way our brain processes this information is similar to how it processes real-life experiences. This can trigger physiological responses that help regulate the nervous system, which means we can call on the memory, the essence, the energetic footprint of someone or something that helps us feel grounded and safe when our nervous systems need a little extra love or care.

I call this process a "soothing recall" and it gives us an opportunity to source safety internally by imagining that we are in a nonjudgmental space, where we feel accepted and valued, with someone who cares for us deeply or would support us fully. In this way, we can create the relational safety that we need to thrive as humans[16]—with the benefit that it is available to us at all times, exactly as we are. Where Emotional Outsourcing would have us do, be, perform, and conform to achieve the sense (however tenuous) that we are unconditionally loved and approved of, soothing recalls require only our own imagination and connect us in with those nervous system resources we spoke about earlier. Even when it is not possible to connect physically with a person we love, just bringing a nurturing parent, pet, plant, or safe place to mind can help us connect with that comfort energetically.[17] For example, I often practice soothing recalls by talking to my long-gone dog, Francis Bacon (she went by Frankie)—the bestest girl ever. A friend of mine's go-to recall is to imagine herself on the balcony of her apartment in Spain, listening to the swallows and sipping a *tinto de verano* while she watches the sky turn purple and gold in the twilight.

You get to choose your safe haven soother: It could be your grandmother who always made you feel cherished, your best friend, a Sesame Street character—anyone or anything that gives you a sense of calm. It could even be a place, like the forest you wandered as a child, or your favorite spot on the beach, the energy of Pachamama or Mother Earth, crystals, animals, and so on. And here's the key—it doesn't matter if they're alive, dead, or geographically far away, or even a character in a book (no reason not to let Mafalda or Mr. Rogers comfort you, right?). A soothing recall is about bringing them into your present moment—imagining what it felt like to be with them, to hear their voice, to feel their warmth or presence in your life. You are resourcing their essence in your mind, and your body will respond.

Whenever my client Brett noticed that she was at a +4 in her nervous system,* she would take a long breath and call up the vision of her *abuela*, bustling around the warm haven of her kitchen. She'd picture herself in her favorite chair by the comal back in Michoacan, nibbling a fresh tortilla and telling her *abuela* her problems, the same way she did as a child: rambling about how a new project at work was keeping her up until 4 a.m., or how her son was failing math, or how worried she was that a friend didn't like her anymore because she hadn't texted her at all since Brett had RSVP'd no to her birthday drinks. When she was finished, she imagined the loving touch of her *abuela*'s weathered hand on her back, that recollection grounding and soothing her now.

Whoever and whatever you call to mind, the key is that it feel as real to you as possible. Fill in the sensory details, noting the temperature of the air, the colors, the aromas, and so forth. If you don't know what to do or what you would need from that person, that's okay. As a starting point, try to imagine that person petting your hair or giving you a hug. If physical contact doesn't feel right, call to mind how they would sound telling you that they love you, or that they will be there to hold you, no matter what happens. You'll know

---

* Remember our nervous system mapping exercise in chapter 3? If you need a refresher on nervous system arousal levels, head back to page 92.

you've found your resource when you notice that you're breathing with more ease and the tension in your body has loosened.

Steps to a Soothing Recall

1. **Orient:** Take just a second to remind your nervous system when and where you are.
2. **Settle into stillness:** Take a slow, deep breath and find a quiet space, either physically or mentally.
3. **Recall them in your mind:** Picture the loved one or energy you feel comforted by—whether they are alive, gone, or distant, a book character or a concept like the wind, rain, or earth. Imagine them with as much sensory detail as possible.
4. **Engage your senses:** Imagine their voice, the way they might speak gently to you. Visualize their comforting presence, the warmth of their hand, or their familiar scent. Let these details fill your body with a sense of calm—you're not alone.
5. **Invite support:** Picture them offering you exactly what you need—whether that's a hug, a reassuring word, or simply being there with you in the moment.
6. **Notice the shift:** Pay attention to your breath and body. Are you breathing more easily? Do you feel less tension? When you sense a softening in your body or feel yourself sigh or yawn, you've tapped into that resource.
7. **Orient:** As always, we end by orienting our nervous systems to the here and now.

These simple steps can bring the calming energy of your loved one into the present, offering your nervous system an anchor of support and safety.

Bonus Resource: Co-regulation

Co-regulation happens when our nervous system attunes to another person, creating an energetic exchange that helps both creatures shift into ventral vagal—feeling safe, secure, and grounded in the moment.[18] It's the process of reciprocating and shaping emotional states with another being. My nervous system influences yours, and yours influences mine—so much so that we can literally change each other's heart rate, breathing, and overall physiology. Think about being scared as a kiddo and curling up next to a calm person or pet—their chill was contagious, their presence a tether to safety. That's the magic of co-regulation. And here's the thing: If you've been emotionally outsourcing, you've been doing this for others for ages—reaching across time, space, and energy to tend to them. The work now is to turn that same care inward. To offer yourself the same steadying presence you so freely give.

A lack of well-attuned, nourishing co-regulation is exactly what Emotional Outsourcing is trying to compensate for. When we lean on codependent, perfectionist, and people-pleasing patterns, we're (unwittingly) trying to secure care, attention, affection, and safety from the people around us—managing their responses so our nervous system can feel just a little safer. And to an extent, it works. But it's hollow.

True co-regulation isn't about earning safety or orchestrating connection—it's a *consensual, intentional* process of creating safety *with* another, the foundation of real interdependence. The more we reach out and allow ourselves to co-regulate, the more our nervous system starts to believe that being with other people—*even and especially* when we're upset, sad, angry, or out of sorts—is not only safe but *available* to us, even if it wasn't in our youth. Because co-regulation isn't just a nice-to-have—it's a vital, biological part of being human.

When we co-regulate, we *consensually* "borrow" someone else's grounded, regulated nervous system—either to help us find our way back into ventral vagal or to feel safe enough to *stay* with our anger, sadness, grief, frustration, or panic and process it within the container their nervous system creates. It's about getting tenderoni so folks can explore their own tenderoni in ways they may never have had the chance to before—which is pretty damn magical indeed.

If the person you've been connecting with in your soothing recalls is physically available to you, they can be an excellent person to reach out to for co-regulation. If not, don't worry. You might equally try reaching out to a member of your chosen family (aka friends), romantic partner, loving family member, therapist, coach, or mental health professional to ask for their support. And don't forget that pets and plants can co-regulate with us too!

Whomever you choose as your co-regulation buddy, the goal is to connect in a way that helps both of you feel more grounded and understood. It starts with really listening to each other—not just hearing the words but getting the whole picture of how someone's feeling, the way they're standing, the look on their face, and the tone of their voice. It's about creating a space where the other person feels like you get them, which can help calm a frazzled nervous system.

When it's okay with both people, a simple touch can make a big difference. A hug, a pat on the back, or just holding hands can make both of you feel more connected and less alone. It's amazing how a small gesture can send waves of calm through your body. Breathing together is another straightforward yet powerful way to sync up with someone. When you both breathe in a slow, steady rhythm, it's like your bodies are saying, "Hey, we're in this together." It's a silent and effective way to help each other relax.

GLIMMERS

Glimmers are my absolute favorites. Introduced to me through Deb Dana's book *Polyvagal Theory in Therapy*, glimmers are moments of joy, lightness, and positivity. They serve as a sort of balm and counterbalance to the sting of triggers—feelings and situations that send our nervous systems zinging down the polyvagal ladder into fight or flight or collapse. Glimmers beckon us back to our window of capacity.[19]

Emotional Outsourcing is often fueled by a scarcity of self-generated positivity. When we don't have an internal well of positive feelings to draw from—whether due to chronic stress, trauma, or simply the habit of placing others' needs before our own—we naturally turn to other people to find the emotional nutrients we require. This lack of internal positivity, and often a lack of positive self-regard, keeps us seeking approval or soothing from external relationships, creating a loop where our sense of well-being hinges on the feelings, opinions, and responses of others. Glimmers, tiny moments of joy or warmth, are an antidote to that. They offer microdoses of positivity that remind us that there's a whole wellspring of joy within, independent of anyone else's actions or approval.

A glimmer is not just something nice or positive; it goes deeper, engaging the nervous system in a way that shifts us toward safety and connection. Glimmers are those subtle sensory moments that signal to our nervous system, particularly to our vagus nerve, that we are safe, grounded, and okay in the world. Unlike a generic positive experience, which might feel mentally pleasant, a glimmer speaks directly to the body's nonverbal cues of safety and regulation. It's like your nervous system taking a little exhale, saying, "Ah, we're good here."

What sets a glimmer apart from something merely nice or positive is how it interacts with the autonomic nervous system. Glimmers activate the parasympathetic system, helping us climb up the polyvagal ladder into a ventral vagal state of connection, calm, and openness. This isn't just a mental acknowledgment of something pleasant but a full-body recognition that we are safe, and that safety allows us to reconnect with joy, curiosity, and playfulness. It's a physiological shift, even if small and subtle, that brings us toward our window of capacity.

For example, while both a warm cup of coffee and a hug can feel "nice," a glimmer goes beyond feeling good in the moment. The hug might regulate your nervous system, settling the heart rate and deepening the breath, sending cues of safety throughout your body. The coffee could be a nice morning ritual that reminds your body of warmth, predictability, and ease. In these moments, your nervous system recognizes cues that bring you out of sympathetic arousal (fight or flight) or dorsal vagal shutdown (collapse) and into a state where you feel safe, connected, and able to engage with the world.

So a glimmer isn't just about external enjoyment; it's an internal, embodied moment where your nervous system shifts, however briefly, toward regulation. Glimmers are especially impactful when they resonate with our inner children, tapping into the parts of ourselves that still carry the unmet needs and desires of our younger selves. Our inner children—those vulnerable, playful, and sometimes wounded parts of us—are often attuned to what brings a sense of comfort, safety, or joy. A glimmer that resonates with these parts is like giving them exactly what they've been longing for, perhaps something they missed out on during their formative years. This could be something as simple as the warmth of sunlight on our skin or as involved as taking yourself to Comic-Con to affirm that nerdy inner kiddo who still longs to feel like she belongs. What your glimmers are doesn't matter and there is no way to get them wrong, so long as they remind a part of you of being held, cared for, or safe, you're doing it right. The resonance happens when a glimmer fulfills a need or brings forth a memory, feeling, or desire that aligns with those core, often undernourished aspects of ourselves.

Think of how a child might respond to a favorite toy or a loving smile—glimmers offer that same kind of nourishment to the inner child, but in the form of subtle sensory or emotional cues in our adult lives. When we encounter something that makes us feel warm, seen, or loved—like that fresh bagel or the scent of santal and juniper—it's not just adult you appreciating the moment. The inner children within us light up, too, because those experiences speak to their need for safety and care. They remind those parts of us that the world can be good, safe, delightful, and nurturing.

When the stress, distress, and trauma of the past makes positivity feel sus or icky, know that you don't have to go all Pollyanna or torch the cool-kid-aloof demeanor that has kept you safe to be able to acknowledge that your human nature is actually to attune to things that make life feel less garbage, which is what glimmers do. You can still be Too Cool For School while allowing these gentle waves of comfort to carry you back to a place of balance and peace.

Accessing glimmers as a resource is about training yourself to notice subtle moments of safety, warmth, and joy that speak to your nervous system. Here's how to cultivate them on purpose:

1. **Engage your senses:** Glimmers work through the body's sensory system. Make a point to slow down and tune in to the moments that might seem banal but that you find pleasant: the smell of fresh laundry, a smile from someone across the room, the light on your kitten's shiny coat. Take time to ask yourself:
    - What do I feel against my skin right now? (The soft fabric of your shirt, a cool breeze on your face?)
    - What smells or sounds are present? (The comforting aroma of cookies in the oven or the soothing rhythm of distant traffic?)

- What do I see that brings ease or even just a neutral okayish feeling? (Perhaps it's the way sunlight filters through leaves or a funny picture that lifts your mood.)

2. **Recall what resonates with your inner children:** Spend a little time remembering younger versions of yourself and what lit them up. Did sixteen-year-old you love the freedom and self-determination of driving around with the windows down and the music blasting? Was seven-year-old you a die-hard Lego enthusiast? Or maybe you loved getting to cook with your auntie. Is there something you can do to call forward those old feelings of love, care, and safety? As a kitten step, engaging in self-soothing or nurturing rituals like playing music you loved as a kid or eating a favorite childhood snack can bring up glimmers that resonate with those unmet needs. And again, if you have no childhood memories or can't access anything nice or lovely, borrow from a book or a film—it's all about the sensation, not having actually for reals done the thing.
3. **Tune in to your body:** Glimmers interact directly with the nervous system, so paying attention to your body's nonverbal cues is key. When you feel something that calms you or gives you a small sense of joy, notice how your body responds. Does your breath deepen? Do your muscles relax? Do you feel a sense of warmth or lightness in your chest? This physiological shift is a hallmark of a glimmer, signaling that your body is moving toward regulation. Over time, you can train your nervous system to recognize these shifts more easily, helping you tune in to what feels grounding and good.

Once you have a list of reliable glimmers, challenge yourself to incorporate them into a daily ritual. For example, on a recent business trip, my client Kate's flight got delayed. Initially, she was frazzled and frustrated after racing around to get to the airport on time, but as she sat at the gate, coffee in hand, she realized it was the first time in years (since becoming a mom) that she'd been able to drink a hot cuppa in peace. It reminded her of quiet Sunday mornings in high school with her dad—just the two of them on the couch, steaming mugs of coffee, while he read the paper. Tearing up at the memory, she realized this was a glimmer she could gift herself more often. So, Kate made a commitment to spend fifteen minutes each morning in solitude, savoring her coffee and that memory of her pops. This commitment might have seemed minor to an outsider, but for Kate, it represented a profound shift. The challenge wasn't in finding the time; it was in granting herself the permission to find comfort and peace in just being.

Kitten Step: Inhale, Hold, Exhale for Support in Dorsal

If you're feeling deeply shut down—disconnected, foggy, heavy, or numb—breathing alone might not feel like enough to pull you back into the present. That's because in a dorsal vagal state, the body has already hit the brakes *hard*—like a phone in low-power mode, conserving energy wherever it can. But even in that slowed-down state, we can send gentle signals to the nervous system that it's safe to shift. One powerful way to do that? A subtle tweak to your breath: *inhale, hold, exhale.*

This technique gives your system a moment to *register* the inhale before releasing it—helping to wake up the body without pushing too hard or fast. It's like a whisper to your nervous system: *Hey, we're here. We're breathing. Let's take our time.*

Here's what I'll invite you to try:

Inhale for 4 counts.

Hold for 2 counts—*just a gentle pause, no forcing.*

Exhale for 6 counts.

Repeat 2 more times for a total of 3 breaths.

Notice how you feel before and after.

That soft hold at the top of the inhale invites a tiny moment of presence, a pause that helps bring just a little more awareness back into your body. The slow exhale still does the heavy lifting of signaling safety, but this little variation can be especially helpful when you feel *too* shut down to engage with the world around you.

And remember, *there's no wrong way to do this.* If your breath is shorter, adjust the numbers—maybe it's inhale for 3, hold for 1, exhale for 5. The goal isn't perfection; it's just to offer your body a different rhythm, a gentle shift toward connection, one breath at a time.

~

Mi amor, the more time you spend in regulation, the more possible regulation becomes. Every time you resource your nervous system with orienting or grounding, each time you do a body scan, have a soothing recall with a loved one, or cultivate your glimmers, you are reminding your body that you're here, you've got this, and adult you can keep you safe. And as your window of capacity slowly but surely widens, the easier it will become to intervene lovingly and choicefully on your own behalf when you need to call yourself home. The trick is to go slowly. Sloooooow, slow slowly. Slower than that. Trauma is "too much too fast too soon," and so for the nervous system, slow is safe, and there is nothing to be gained by forcing your way through these practices.

Remember, sweetling, you spent decades entraining one way of being safe into your nervous system. It's not going to stop doing its best to keep you alive just because you read a cool book and decided you're safe now. Be gentle, go slowly, and give yourself grace. Don't forget all that great work around self-compassion and self-talk that you learned back in chapter 5! It all works together.

Additional Somatic Resources

My love, there are truly so many wonderful ways to resource our nervous systems. The five I've outlined in this chapter—orienting, grounding, body scan, soothing recall, and glimmers—are like your starter pack. These are the five that will get you started on your journey to lovingly support your nervous system into regulation. However, I would be very, very remiss if I didn't mention two additional somatic resources: dance and psychedelics.

A 2024 study in the *BMJ* (formerly the *British Medical Journal*) showed that dancing was more effective than any depression treatment currently available—including SSRIs or antidepressant drugs. Yes, *just* dancing, with no other interventions.[20] Of course, this is not news to Indigenous cultures, whose brilliance recognized centuries ago that movement, especially in community, is profound medicine. Through movement we can achieve emotional release, become more aware of our bodies, and have tremendously positive impacts on our mental health.

Psychedelic work, when done with care and intention in a legal, well-facilitated context, of course, offers an opportunity for healing that spans beyond the cognitive mind and reaches the deepest layers of our spiritual and biological being. On a biological level, psychedelics like psilocybin and MDMA help reduce activity in the brain's default mode network (DMN), the part responsible for self-referential thinking and rumination. For those of us who live in Emotional Outsourcing, where we constantly manage others' needs at the expense of our own, the DMN often becomes an echo chamber of negative self-talk and anxiety over others' expectations. By loosening its grip, psychedelic work loosens the DMN's rigid, habitual patterns, offering space for the mind to explore new ways of being and rewrite old narratives.[21] Psychedelics calm the hypervigilance of the sympathetic nervous system, allowing us to drop into more restorative states, giving the body and mind a chance to experience safety in a way that feels new and expansive.

JOURNAL PROMPTS
HOW TO SIT WITH A FEELING

One of the things I hear most from coaching clients is that they don't know how to sit with their feelings. And that's so normal, my perfect peppermint patty! After all, you spent most of your life teaching yourself to do the exact opposite for your own protection. That said, being able to accompany ourselves through the breadth of human emotions is vital stuff. We can't resolve the somatic roots of our Emotional Outsourcing unless we learn to navigate challenging feelings with grace; moreover, we can't handle in others what we can't handle in ourselves, my love, so unless and until you can sit with your own anger, sadness, disappointment, frustration, or discomfort, you will continue to control, fix, people-please, et cetera, to avoid the distress of watching others experience those emotions (hellooooo, Emotional Outsourcing). So, my love, let's take a moment together to unpack this process and practice sitting with our feelings together.

Big picture, being with an emotion means being able to know and feel whatever feelings are true for you in that moment without getting fully overwhelmed by them. Through a process of mindful acceptance and self-regulation, you can experience intense emotions of all sorts from a safe, cozy seat in your window of capacity. This takes time, practice, and lots of repetition, and typically follows the same handful of steps:

1. **Orient, orient, orient!:** Always start by bringing your nervous system into the here and now by simply looking around and reminding your mind and body of when and where you are.

2. **Ground yourself:** Use grounding techniques to stay present and centered. This can include sensory experiences like touching a piece of fabric, smelling a favorite scent, or listening to calming music, which can help anchor you in the present moment. Keep orienting and grounding as needed—the more the merrier!

3. **Acknowledge the emotion:** Start by looking inward to notice and name the feeling you are experiencing in this moment. This could be anger, despair, fear, shame, joy, overwhelm, pride, vulnerability,

ebullience, and so on. Having a feelings wheel like the one available at beatrizalbina.com/feelingswheel might help you name your emotions with greater specificity. You don't have to name them perfectly because "perfect" doesn't even exist here. This is about Being With, not cataloging. Let yourself get it more or less right and move on.

4. **Pause and breathe:** As you name the emotion with a statement (aloud or internal) like "I notice that I am feeling ________," take a deep breath, focusing on the long, slow exhale.

5. **Observe without judgment:** Pay attention to where you feel the emotion in your body, if you feel it. Note any sensations associated with the emotion (tightness, warmth, pressure, etc.) without judging or trying to change them.

6. **Get curious:** Leading with a desire to understand, and *not* a desire to shift the feeling, ask yourself what message the emotion might be conveying. What might it need? Don't get discouraged if you don't hear, feel, or know an answer right away, or even the first several times you practice sitting. Curiosity is, itself, healing.

7. **Honor the feeling:** Accept the emotion as a part of your current experience, without trying to suppress or ignore it, which can be wicked challenging at first! Acceptance doesn't mean you resign yourself to the feeling, or even that you "approve" of it. This is an opportunity to validate your real experience and treat yourself with compassion, getting real that this is what you are truly feeling in the moment.

8. **Follow the feeling:** If your anger wants you to push on a wall, push. If your sadness wants you to crawl under the covers and bawl, let yourself. As long as you're not harming yourself or others, follow the impulse of your emotion. When we allow our nervous system to move the energy of a feeling *all the way through*—instead of resisting or suppressing it—it's shocking how briefly it actually lasts. Most of my clients are stunned to realize that when they stop pushing their emotions down and simply let them take up space for a moment, they move through so much faster.

9. **Reflect and respond:** Once you've let it out and feel more regulated, spend some time journaling about the emotion that came up and what it expressed to you, and reflecting on what may have prompted that feeling. Focus on being with yourself and holding space for whatever came and comes up without judgment. Do an Anchor Scan to orient as you come to a close.

If, as you move through these steps, your emotion feels too overwhelming to manage alone, seek co-regulating support from a friend, family member, pet, or mental health professional. Sharing your feelings and experiences can provide relief and additional perspectives on how to cope and is a natural, healthy way to lean into that interdependence we're working toward.

Ultimately, the goal is integration: bringing the insights you've gained from experiencing and reflecting on your emotions into a broader sense of yourself, your patterns, and your needs so you can be with yourself fully and with those you love interdependently.

Chapter 7

The Thought Work Protocol

Picture this: Ever since the layoffs last year, you've been doing three people's jobs just to keep your understaffed department afloat, and all the extra work has really been taking a toll. You can't remember the last time you had a date night or hung out with a friend, long hours in front of the computer are making your migraines worse, and your anxiety is through the roof. You never let anyone see the cracks and your work is flawless, but after a diagnosis of walking pneumonia and *keep right on walking*, you realize it may be time to talk to your boss about your workload.

You send a carefully worded email at 4 p.m., laying out your current responsibilities and asking for a meeting tomorrow to discuss getting you some support. You wait for a reply, obsessively refreshing your inbox. Twenty minutes pass. Nothing. Heart racing, palms sweaty, you start to pace around your home office. *Did I mess up? Was that too much? I knew it was too much. Why complain? Everyone is overworked. I should just be able to handle this.* Forty minutes (and a full desk re-org) later, nothing. By 9 p.m., still no response, and you're in a full-blown spiral. *Am I going to get fired? What if my boss hates me now? What am I going to do when I see her at the office tomorrow?* Too overwhelmed at the thought of a confrontation, you mark yourself "working from home" to avoid your boss, never mentioning your email or following up to put time on the calendar. The next week, you feel on the verge of a nervous breakdown, yet you said yes to being a colleague's out-of-office contact while they're on parental leave.

Too many of us race through life without pausing to understand what's driving our choices and our actions. Especially when we're mired in our Emotional Outsourcing patterns, we act without discernment, detached from our intuition, and become frustrated when we find ourselves in situations where everyone's needs are met but our own; everyone is pleased except us. But what if, instead of reacting on autopilot, you could pause, take a breath, and notice that the story you're telling yourself in that moment may not be exactly what's happening?

The Thought Work Protocol is the tool I teach to help my clients do just that and get back into the driver's seat of their lives. By pausing to actively engage with our thought patterns, we get to slow that proverbial roll just enough to decide if we actually like how we're living or not. In this chapter, I'm going to show you how to change your habitual thinking step-by-step using the protocol. As you become more aware of your thought habits, you'll be able to create space to respond choicefully to your life, instead of reacting from the past and its long-armed projections, and can write a new script for your life—one that steps out of those codependent, perfectionist, people-pleasing stories for good.

THE POWER OF THE THINK-FEEL-ACT CYCLE

The great neurologist, psychologist, and Holocaust survivor Viktor E. Frankl is often quoted as saying, "Between stimulus and response, there is a space. In that space is our power to choose our response. In our response lies our growth and our freedom."[1] While there's no solid evidence that he said it exactly this way, I include it because the space he (maybe) describes is *exactly* what we cultivate in thought work—and it's central to healing from Emotional Outsourcing, whether Dr. Frankl actually said it or not.

Most of the time, we move through our lives on autopilot. We nod along with the group even if we don't agree. We beat ourselves up when something isn't exactly right without ever really deciding to do so. We don't speak up when our family members say things that hurt us (but we complain the second they're out of the room). We go back on our boundaries, overfunction, overeat, or overexercise, doomscroll, overthink—actions we don't like but we can't seem to shake.

Yet, my love, the reality is that our circumstances don't dictate our actions. There is a process that happens in our minds at lightning speed that determines the way we show up with ourselves, with the world, and in our relationships. That process is summed up as the think-feel-act cycle—a shorthand phrase I use to describe the relationship between our interpretations of the world, the feelings our interpretations bring up (emotions as well as bodily sensations), and what we do as a result. Understanding the think-feel-act cycle is essential to overcoming our Emotional Outsourcing habits, so let's break this down together.

Thoughts are patterned sentences in our minds, our default interpretations based on the past. They're the stories we carry and the meaning we make of our world. We have thousands of thoughts a day, which represent our ideas, opinions, and beliefs and the perspectives that inform our point of view in any situation.[2] Our thoughts reflect everything that we've absorbed from our caregivers, our social environments, and our lived experiences. Over time, the thoughts we have more frequently become neural grooves in our brains. The more often we interpret a situation the same way (i.e., have the same thought about it), the deeper that groove gets and the more likely our brain is to follow down that path. In psychology we call these "heuristics," or mental shortcuts. They're the things that we believe and notice most often in our lives. In Emotional Outsourcing, we get stuck in heuristics like these:

- I'm not enough.
- I'm not worthy of their love.
- I have to earn love and care and rest.
- If I don't do everything, nothing will get done (and that matters because what I get done means something about me).
- I and my house/kids/dinner/career/relationship/everything need to be perfect or I'm a failure.
- If I tell them how I feel, they'll abandon me.
- My feelings are too big/too much.
- If they aren't praising me, then they must hate me.

All these thoughts feed our codependent, perfectionist, people-pleasing actions. You may think this sounds a lot like what we talked about in chapter 2, and you'd be right: The self-stories we learned in childhood become some of our strongest heuristics, our most common thoughts and go-to interpretations of life.

Feelings are sensations in our bodies. They're the racing heart, the clammy hands, the nausea, and the lightness that come from how our nervous system reacts to our thoughts and surroundings, based in our history. We then put words to those physical sensations to describe our experience, for example, anxious, glad, happy, afraid. Our thoughts tell us what meaning to make of the feeling we're having. For example, the sensation of butterflies in your stomach could equally mean that you're excited for a date or that you're nervous about a presentation.

Together, our thoughts and our feelings motivate our **actions**—what you do, or don't do, in a given situation. In this framework, the action you take follows directly from your thoughts and feelings, even if you aren't aware of them, and that's precisely why getting in touch with our think-feel-act cycle is so important. Unless and until we can change our underlying thoughts, we are going to (subconsciously) create the same outcomes for ourselves: exhaustion, anxiety, depression, lopsided relationships, self-abandonment, chronic nervous system dysregulation, and so on.

I want to emphasize, my darlings, that the think-feel-act cycle is most often a subconscious process. And necessarily so! Our neural grooves are the reason you can effortlessly, automatically hug a friend when you see them. You don't have to be aware of the thought "I missed my friend—I'm so happy to see them," and the subsequent feelings of warmth and softness in your limbs when you see them; you just give them a hug hello. The goal of the Thought Work Protocol—and its magic—is that it helps us to slow down so that we can examine our experience of our lives when it's suboptimal and we want change. When we pause to write down our habitual thoughts, feelings, and actions, we give ourselves a chance to notice—and change, where necessary—the interpretations that keep us stuck in Emotional Outsourcing.

Friendly Reminder: Not All Your Thoughts Are Yours

Lovebug, as you dive into the Thought Work Protocol, I want you to do so with the awareness that not all of your thoughts are yours. As we saw in earlier chapters, the thoughts grooved into your adult brain about your role, worth, body, identities, family, and relationships did not spring forth whole from a font of universal truth: They're the earworm chorus of the songs you heard growing up, sung by personal experiences and the larger societal symphony.

Getting to know our think-feel-act cycle is about taking accountability for the thoughts that we're living from, not blaming ourselves for thinking in ways that kept us safe. Self-knowledge and accountability are the bedrock of change, and seeing for yourself what thoughts are running the show gives you the opportunity to approach your life with choice and intention.

THE THOUGHT WORK PROTOCOL

While the physical process of reprogramming neural pathways is pretty darn complex and involves things like the modulation of synaptic strength, changes in neurotransmitter release, and the growth of new dendrites and axons, the experience of it in our minds isn't nearly so complicated: We do something called *Thought Work* to understand and consistently shift our habitual interpretations of the world. Before we can create a new script for our minds, we need to build awareness of what's already happening. The protocol that I teach my clients—and use myself to this day!—is based on cognitive behavioral theory and invites us to reflect on five components of our experience:

- **Observation:** What is the bare-bones, court-admissible, no-adjectives version of this situation that anyone can observe?
- **Interpretation:** What are my automatic thoughts? What meaning am I making?
- **Feeling:** What bodily sensations and emotions are coming up for me?
- **Actions:** What did or didn't I do in response to my interpretation and feelings?
- **Result:** What was the outcome of those actions/inactions in my own life?

In the next few pages, we're going to explore each part of the protocol step-by-step, and you're going to want your journal handy as we begin this work. Even though it can be tempting to do thought work in your mind, the protocol works best when we write it all down in black and white for ourselves. Taking that extra time to jot it down will allow you to track that think-feel-act cycle with more objectivity, which in turn will help you to observe your thought habits with less judgment. If you'd prefer a structured worksheet to guide you, you'll find one in appendix B or on www.beatrizalbina.com/book.

Story Follows State

We nervous system nerds love to say "story follows state." In other words, the meaning we make about what's happening in a given moment is tremendously impacted by the state of our nervous system. Remember back in chapter 3, where we learned that when we're regulated, all the parts of our brains are working as an integrated whole, with the cortex (logic center) and amygdala (emotion center) engaged with each other as a team as best they can; however, when we leave that window of capacity, the parts of our brain responsible for taking in new information, communicating our needs, connecting with others, and problem solving effectively go offline, as it were.[3] Furthermore, when our nervous systems are no longer predominantly in ventral vagal, our cognitive capacity diminishes, as the brain shifts from thoughtful, nuanced processing to survival mode, prioritizing threat detection over complex reasoning, problem solving, or creativity. As a result, your nervous system state quite literally limits the thoughts you may have access to in a given moment, and you can't think so well when you're trying to not be someone's lunch, like when you're in functional freeze like we tend to be in Emotional Outsourcing.

This is why we always start with somatic work. Trying to do thought work with a dysregulated nervous system is like pushing a grocery store cart with one wheel locked: You're gonna get frustrated, and you're also not gonna get very far.

So here's my caution: Don't fall into the trap of approaching thought work as a substitute for somatic practices. It may feel more comfortable to privilege the brain over the body and to intellectualize our feelings instead of feeling them (especially if your body is holding a couple of decades of repressed rage-fear-grief-sadness-oppression). I know. I've been there, too, and it's a *lot* to unpack, hold, and process without wanting to run for the hills. Even so, if you want to shift your experience of yourself and your relationships, if you want to feel more physically and emotionally well, and you want all that hard work to become lasting change, you get to do both, my love—thought work *and* somatic work—they both matter.

Observation

The first step of the Thought Work Protocol is to describe without any adjectives, storytelling, embellishment, or assumptions the shortest possible version of what is happening in the moment. Sounds simple enough, but in practice it can be very challenging to separate the court-admissible, observable facts of a situation from the story we're telling about it.

The trouble is, most of us believe that our interpretation of life is actually the 100 percent true and real, unchangeable facts. Our thoughts and emotions come in to color our experience so quickly that many people don't realize the difference between "She went rogue and trashed our whole slide deck, and now we have nothing to show to the partners!" and "My colleague made changes to a shared document without consulting the team," or we believe our story that

"He's such a jerk!" when the fact is "He said words" and you actually get to decide how you want to think about those situations.

Thanks to neuroception (the way your young nervous system encoded situations as either safe or unsafe) and the meaning-making machinery of our minds, we're quick to treat *our* reality based on our projections and heuristics as the only possible reality, and so we react to life the way we always have, instead of finding choicefulness or agency to decide how we want to think and feel. In thought work we pause and give ourselves space to notice that how you experience something is not necessarily the same thing as what happened and is definitely not the only way you can think about the situation at hand.

A useful observation is the most neutral explanation of what you can see about the situation at hand. When you start the Thought Work Protocol, bring to mind the circumstance or situation that you want to explore, and peel it *all* the way down to its facts. You're just going for the plot—no extras, emotions, or assumptions.

- *My mom is always on my case about working out. Am I really that fat? Why can't she leave me alone! I hate this!*
    - Observation: My mom comments on my weight three or four times a month.

- *How could Harper have gotten such a bad score? Her future is going to be ruined if she doesn't get these grades up, and I'll look like a failure in front of my friends!*
    - Observation: Harper got a 78 on her math test.

- *He's always on his phone and ignoring me when I talk to him!*
    - Observation: John uses his phone during dinner every night.

- *There goes my sister again, posting vacation photos from God knows where while I'm stuck here taking care of Dad, day after day, because I'm not a selfish brat like her.*
    - Observation: My sister shared a picture from her vacation.

The easiest way to tell if you've gotten to that neutral, facts-only observation is to check if there are any adjectives. If there are, take a breath and ask yourself what a stranger would be able to notice if they walked into a freeze-frame of the situation. *Yes, I, too, can see that there are dishes in the sink. Yes, I, too, can confirm that it is currently 4:45 p.m. and Suzy does not have her shoes on.* Once you're clear on your observation, write it down in your journal.

Interpretation

The interpretation section of the Thought Work Protocol is where we get really honest with ourselves about the automatic, default stories we're telling and our nervous system state. In your journal, you'll write a one- to two-sentence statement that gets right to the heart of your interpretation of the moment—the most potent belief, perception, or fear that informs the meaning your brain has made. For example, you text a friend, and they don't respond for hours. At first, it's just a fact—your message sits unread. But then, the thoughts start rolling in: *Did I say something weird? Are they mad at me? They must not care about me as much as I care about them.* And suddenly, your interpretation is *"I'm too much,"* or *"People always leave,"* or *"I have to work to keep people close."* Or let's say you receive a surprise calendar invite from your boss, subject line "15-min chat." Those instant racing thoughts of "Sh*t sh*t sh*t, what happened? Did I do something wrong?" suggest that your interpretation is "I'm in trouble" (and that it's probably a very young inner child speaking!).

Now, before you get frustrated by your knee-jerk interpretations, remember that they're not personal failings—they're part of your heuristic neural programming. Nervous system nerds like to say that "story follows state in the nervous system"—meaning that the state you're in directly impacts the thoughts available to you. When you're regulated (ventral vagal), your thoughts tend to be curious, open, and trusting. When you're in sympathetic activation (fight/flight), those same thoughts may morph into catastrophizing, blame, or hypervigilance—"I have to" thoughts. If you've dropped into dorsal shutdown, your thoughts may turn toward hopelessness, self-doubt, or a sense that nothing matters—"I can't" thoughts.

I like to use the metaphor of an old-school library card catalog to explain how our nervous system shapes our thoughts. Imagine three main drawers—one for safety (ventral vagal), one for fight or flight (sympathetic), and one for shutdown (dorsal). Whichever drawer your nervous system accesses determines the default set of thoughts available to you. When you're regulated, the cards are filled with curiosity, self-trust, and connection. But when you're in survival mode, the only thoughts you can pull are ones about danger, urgency, or hopelessness. Your brain doesn't create a neutral narrative; it pulls from whatever drawer your nervous system has opened. This is why I encourage you to name the nervous system state you're in and track your arousal level—it gives you profound insight into how your habitual thoughts shift depending on your physiological state.

And for humans with infradian rhythms (aka, those with menstrual cycles), hormonal fluctuations also shape the thoughts available to us. Estrogen and progesterone influence neurotransmitters like oxytocin, serotonin, dopamine, and GABA, which means that depending on where you are in your cycle, you may experience more optimism and motivation—or more self-doubt and sensitivity.[4] Just like nervous system state determines which "drawer" of thoughts you can pull from, hormonal shifts can change which cards are even in the drawer that day.*

By identifying both your emotional state and your nervous system state, you'll start to recognize the patterns—how your thoughts and feelings shift with your arousal level and which interpretations are more likely to show up in different states. This awareness is key because it helps you catch state-dependent thinking before it dictates your actions. Instead of believing every thought at face value, you can pause and ask: *Is this thought coming from a regulated place? Or is this my nervous system reacting to a perceived threat?* This is how we start to untangle old patterns and reclaim our agency.

You'll know you've found the interpretation or story that is fueling your feelings because it makes you go *oof!* when you read it. Often, to get there, we have to get curious about our stories and ask, "What's under that?" For example, most arguments are rarely about what they seem to be about in the moment. Sure, on the surface you're yelling at your partner because they forgot to pick up milk or do the dishes like they promised, but under that is anger about doing all the emotional and invisible labor in the household, and how invalidated and overlooked that makes you feel, plus that lingering childhood wounding from never feeling seen or respected. Your observation is that the dishes are still in the sink, and the interpretation you write in your protocol is, "I don't matter to you or you would do the dishes." You may have to ask yourself, "What's under that?" three, four, even five times before you get all the way to the bottom.

---

* Just because a thought is influenced by hormonal shifts doesn't make it any less real or important to work with—your nervous system and brain are still experiencing it as truth. And yet, people socialized as women are taught to over-control and under-experience our own feelings and lives, dismissing what we feel as *just hormones* rather than recognizing it as meaningful data. Instead of writing off these thoughts, we get to meet them with curiosity, compassion, and the same intentional thought work we'd apply to any other state-dependent belief.

It's possible to have multiple interpretations of a scenario. However, for the purposes of the protocol, we always work with one thought or story at a time. You can always do more protocols, my love—but take each interpretation one thought at a time.

Get It All Out

Distilling an interpretation is often easier after we've let ourselves have *all* of our thoughts. One of the most time-honored habits of Emotional Outsourcing is keeping it all bottled up inside, hiding our thoughts and feelings from ourselves and the world, pretending we're okay, and stuffing it down, down, down until we don't feel anything and have no clue what we're actually thinking. Giving yourself free rein and a safer space to get it all out of your head and your heart—knowing that nothing you say is "wrong" or permanent and that you will not judge yourself for what you say—can have surprising emotional and physical benefits. Inspired by the work of John Sarno, MD, and his protégée Nicole Sachs, LCSW, who pioneered the expressive writing technique,[5] I often encourage my clients to begin with what I like to call a Fire Write.

To do this, set a timer for 2–5 minutes, call to mind the whole story, and give yourself permission to say anything and everything you need to. Mean, vile, frightening, embarrassing, improper, shameful, irrational—whatever you're keeping bottled up? Let it flow. Once you've ladled out some of your emotional reservoir onto the page (to borrow an image from Sachs's work),[6] read it over and choose one interpretation that feels most true, and write it down in your Thought Work Protocol.

Let me give you an example. My client Liza was ready to breathe fire. She'd seen the workout clothes she bought her twenty-year-old daughter, Beth, as a birthday gift crumpled in a box labeled "donations" in Beth's car, the tags still on. In her journal, she wrote:

> *Why is Beth always like this! I told her she needed to start working out and I even bought her all those expensive clothes...and with all I've suffered and done and given up for her! Can't she just do this one thing? Just like her brother and her father, she doesn't care about how I feel, she doesn't care if I'm upset, she doesn't respect my hard work, she doesn't respect the nice things I get her, she doesn't respect me, she doesn't care about finding a good husband, she doesn't care about her health, she doesn't care about what people will think about me and the family if she's not fit, she has no respect for this family, what will people think of me if she's not fit and married? I can't bear the thought of being the mom of just another fat American kid. I do so much for her and she can't just do this one thing for me! It's for her own good! Why can't she just listen?! And why am I the bad guy because I get upset that she's not taking care of herself?! Why do I even bother!*

I call the stories that come up during these Fire Writes *process thoughts*: the free-flowing stories that exist in our minds before we refine them and get to the root of those stories. Process thoughts are a gold mine of interpretations to bring to our thought work. Seeing your full story there on the page often points the way to the interpretation that is driving your feelings and actions. For example, if Liza were to start from her process thoughts and ask, "What's under that?" that might sound like:

- *What's under that?* So much frustration!! I just don't understand why she can't take better care of herself!
- *What's under that?* I took care of her for decades! I did everything for her! I *still* do everything for her!

- *What's under that?* I'm so jealous because she has what I never had: No one takes care of me.
- *What's under that?* I'm sad that I put so much effort into everyone else and don't feel cared for in my own life—I'm resentful and angry.
- *What's under that?* I'm scared that when I'm old I won't be able to take care of myself anymore and nobody will be there to take care of me.

Ah. There it is. By staying with it and digging deeper, Liza can go from the surface story, "My daughter is so ungrateful!" to the interpretation, "I'm scared I won't be cared for when I'm old."

So why do I call them Fire Writes? Because when we get started it can be helpful to destroy our work once it's done, as a way to let our nervous systems know it's safe to experience it all—no one can find our writing and come for us. Feel free to burn.

Feeling

Feelings are the emotions and physical sensations that arise as the immediate results of our interpretive thought. Sometimes our feelings are obvious to us and sometimes we have to give ourselves permission to look inward and get curious. For purposes of the Thought Work Protocol, we want to keep it simple, so your mission (should you choose to accept it!) is to write down the one primary feeling that your interpretation creates and whatever sensations arise.

I notice that my clients are often quick to race over the physical sensations, and I urge you, my darling, to pause and listen in to your body. A feeling is a conscious interpretation of an emotion (e.g., boredom, frustration, happiness, calm, peace, annoyance, joy), accompanied by physical sensations in the body (e.g., buzzing, tightness, nausea, pain, lightness). You know by now that the state of our nervous system is foundational to our experience of the world. When we neglect to listen to our body fully, it's easy to miss the impact that our thoughts are having on our actions, and how that plays out more broadly in our lives.

Now, my perfectionist peonies, please remember that there is no "right" way to answer the question "What am I feeling?" We're not interested in what you're *supposed* to feel, or what your friend feels, or what you would like to feel. Whatever is true for you in the moment is the most useful information for you. If you're struggling to tap into feelings, that's okay. Consider looking to a feelings wheel like the free resource available at beatrizalbina.com/feelingswheel to help you name your emotions, and I recommend using the Nervous System Arousal Levels and Tracker on page 92 and in appendix A as a support for connecting physical sensations and nervous system states.

Action

It can be challenging to be honest about the things we do on autopilot that we aren't exactly proud of, like losing it on the people we love the most or yelling at customer service folks instead of our partners because the phone rep is safer to call out; saying nasty things to and about ourselves; going against our own values or breaking promises; and a thousand other actions (and inactions—like procrastinating or not exercising) that be so *ughhhhh* to admit to, even to ourselves. Our brains whisper, *Don't look behind that curtain!* focusing on the people around us and what *they* did to buffer against the discomfort of accountability, to see where we can transfer out the rage and annoyance, the guilt and shame we feel inside. I mean, sure—your husband stormed out . . . but only after you told him that he was useless and you don't know why you bother to ask for help if he's just going to disappoint you. And listen, I get it—owning our messiest moments isn't exactly a party. But if we *don't* look behind that curtain, we stay stuck playing the same role in the same tired script. And honestly? If we're going to be doing all this emotional labor anyway, we might as well put in for a promotion.

One sneaky place to look for our action is what we *didn't* do in a situation. Check in on that negative space and get just as curious about where you froze or defaulted to inaction as a result of your thoughts and feelings. For example, my client Geetarani often had the experience of people mispronouncing her name. The idea of correcting anyone made her palms sweat, and after years of nicknames and bumbling teachers, she carried the story that her name was just too hard to pronounce so she shouldn't expect her white colleagues to know better (thank you, internalized white-settler colonialism). So when her boss called her "Ronnie" again, even though she hated it, she didn't bother correcting him. That inaction—"Didn't speak up about mispronouncing my name"—is, in this case, her action that she can put into the Thought Work Protocol to work with.

Result

The final step of the protocol is to ask yourself what the outcome of your actions was for your own life. I'm going to say that again, my love, because it's super important: In this protocol, we are only interested in the result for and in *your* life and *only your life*. Not your partner's, friend's, child's, or colleague's life. Just yours. How did that action turn out for *you*?

I often see clients who are new to the protocol writing down a result like "They stormed off" or "She didn't call me back and she totally hates me now!" or "My mom started crying," but, my sweetest snickerdoodle, while those may be things that happened, none of those outcomes happened *in your own life*. As we practice taking accountability for how our interpretations, nervous system state, and actions all contribute to our own experience of our own life, I invite you, again, to go slow and to focus inward. Offer yourself the attention that you habitually give to others and ask, bravely, "How did this play out for *me*?" The goal is not more rugged individualism and self-focused navel-gazing wellness-culture crapola—no, thank you. The goal is to focus on the one person whose think-feel-act cycle we can control, which is ourselves. And once we understand our own motivation and behavior, we can take responsibility that is ours to take, and nothing more than what is ours—wildly new experiences for most of us!

So instead of "Action: I screamed; Result: She cried," you might write, "Result: I strengthened the neural groove that tells me being angry hurts other people so I shouldn't be angry." Or, instead of "Action: I asked for help; Result: The jerk told me no," you might write, "Result: While I didn't get what I wanted, I was proud of myself for asking for what I needed."

As you can see from these examples, not all results are external. Often, the real impact of our thoughts, feelings, and actions is felt internally. We strengthen or weaken beliefs; we have new feelings—outcomes that live in our minds and hearts, rather than out in the world.

In a rude little twist of life, many of my clients are also surprised to see that the result is precisely the outcome they were trying to avoid, the product of their interpretation of the situation. For example, my client Mathilde wanted to feel more connected to her friend Ben. She knew Ben was grieving the loss of his mother, and Mathilde could never seem to find the right words to talk with him about it. She thought that if she said the wrong thing she'd make it worse, and then she wouldn't know what to say next, and it would all just be so unbearably uncomfortable. It kicked up that familiar functional freeze; buzzing and brain fog would take over and she'd avoid the topic while they were together, then ruminate on how Ben must hate her and feel so let down by her silence, worried about how she could ever face him again. In this case, the result in Mathilde's life is that she feels more distant from her friend. See how that was exactly the opposite of what she wanted? The gift of doing the protocol is that Mathilde was able to see the result she created for herself and to work backward to create a new outcome that was more fulfilling.

~

I know there are a lot of parts, my love, so let's look at an example of how the Thought Work Protocol comes together. My client April grew up in a predominantly white, middle-class community where the value of being "nice" was drilled into her from an early age and she avoided conflict at all costs. When a friend or partner was upset, April would swoop in to offer advice, smooth things over, or take responsibility for everyone's emotional climate (def without listening or checking in). If someone said something hurtful, she was quick to minimize her own emotions, telling herself, *It's no big deal* or *I'm probably overreacting*—which is precisely what happened one afternoon while she and her boyfriend were planning a date night. April wanted to go to the art museum. It was one of her favorite places, and somewhere she had been wanting to share with her partner. She knew it was risky, but she floated it anyway. "Hey, babe, what if we went to the art museum? They do special tours on Saturday and it could be really fun!"

"Uh," her boyfriend stalled, "I was kinda thinking we could go to the game? I don't really do art. It always seemed kinda lame." Stung by his comment but a Good Girl to the core, April shoved down the flood of shame and annoyance, agreeing to go to the game even as, internally, she lamented that they never did what she wanted to do. The next week on our coaching call, we worked through the Thought Work Protocol together:

Observation (bare-bones, court-admissible facts, no adjectives or adverbs): *I asked my boyfriend to go to the art museum; he didn't say that he* ***wanted*** *to go, so instead, we went to a basketball game.*

Interpretation (reactions, automatic thoughts; what meaning am I making? what story am I telling? nervous system state): *I can't do what I want unless the other person is totally on board and it's up to me to ensure they're on board, and even though he didn't say he doesn't want to go to the museum, I don't want to risk him having a bad time and it being my fault. If he's not enthusiastic, I'll feel exposed, like I'm asking for too much, like I'm needy. If I push for what I want, I could be rejected or dismissed, and I'd rather abandon my own desires than feel that sting. Nervous system response: Dorsal vagal (collapsed, shut down, defeated).*

Feeling (emotion, then physical sensations): *resentment—hot cheeks, heavy limbs, fogginess, with tingling in my hands.*

Actions (what you did/didn't do): *I interpreted his lack of enthusiasm for my plan to mean he didn't want to do it; I projected my fears that I don't matter onto him; from my people-pleasing habits I decided to do what I felt he wanted more than what I wanted even though he didn't say no to my plan: Agreed to go to the game despite wanting to go to the museum; smiled and acted like it wasn't a big deal; minimized my own feelings; ruminated afterward about how they never do what I want; avoided bringing up my disappointment later.*

Result (what was the outcome of those actions in *your* life?): *I declined to go to the art museum because my boyfriend said words. I prioritized my boyfriend's interests over my own, reinforced the belief that my interests never matter, felt more distant from myself and him, reinforced* *a dorsal response, missed an opportunity to advocate for myself, created distance with myself.*

Now April has some clarity about what happens in these moments and can start to plan how she'll take care of herself differently in the future, which we'll lay out here *en un momentito.*

When You Get Stuck: Taller Toddler Reminder

It takes courage and thoughtfulness to confront your own stories, feelings, and habitual actions—it is brave work to see how you participate in creating your own experience of your life. If you get stuck or you're struggling, I want to remind you to check in with your body. My love! You are a Taller Toddler and need to treat yourself now like you would like your two- to four-year-old self to be treated. Are you tired? Dehydrated? Hungry? Angry? Overcaffeinated? Hungover? If your body needs some loving attention, pause the protocol, get up, and take care of the basics before getting complicated. Once you've had some water and a nice protein snack, gone to the bathroom, or taken a little walk around the neighborhood, try again.

If you're still really, really stuck in this protocol, start from the thought *I'm stuck.* Like so many of our stories, we believe that the statement "I'm stuck" or "I'm bad at this" or "Thought work doesn't work for me" is a fact, rather than the result of your current thoughts, feelings, and actions combined with your somatic reality. You might be surprised by how thought work around your feelings of stuckness can, in fact, get you unstuck *and* let you practice the protocol. How's that for efficiency?!

HOW TO SHIFT YOUR EXPERIENCE

While you're first getting the hang of it, the Thought Work Protocol serves as a kind of postmortem on your experiences. You notice a moment of shutdown or activation during the day, or your Watcher has been highlighting some common themes lately, and you spend time in your journal the next day to try to understand yourself better.

But thought work isn't just about looking backward—it's also about shaping what comes next. Once we start seeing our patterns clearly, we can use that awareness proactively. This is where an intentional Thought Work Protocol comes in. Instead of just reflecting on past moments, we can prepare for future ones—choosing ahead of time how we want to respond so we can shift our outcomes.

The real gift of thought work is that it helps us in two key ways: to break free from painful thought loops in the moment and to prepare ourselves for situations where we might fall back into old habits. We can decide ahead of time how we want to show up—how we'll shift our responses to create different results in our lives. As long as we're reacting from habit—overfunctioning, buffering, ruminating, shutting down—we'll keep experiencing the same patterns, same frustrations, same outcomes. An intentional Thought Work Protocol gives us a chance to pause between stimulus and response, to step out of autopilot and into choice. It's a gift—not just to our minds, but to our nervous systems—offering us the possibility of something new, so let's learn about it.

Once you have your Thought Work Protocol written out, you get to ask yourself: Do I like this outcome or result? Do I like the experience of my life that I'm creating with the interpretation I'm rockin'? Do I want to keep living this way or do I want to make a change? The most beautiful thing about realizing that your thoughts are not facts is this: You don't have to believe everything you think. Part of becoming an emotional adult is to recognize that you get to choose whether a thought serves you, whether it's accurate, and whether you would like to keep it. Creating an intentional protocol is all about discerning what interpretation will lead you toward the result you desire in your own life and taking those kitten steps to create a new neural groove. If you do decide that you want to make a change, there are three steps we take to build an intentional protocol.

Step 1: Be with What Is

It's normal to get excited about changing what you don't like and Overhauling Your Whole Life, but our brains and bodies work slowly. So our first step when we want to change our interpretation is *not* to dive headlong into a Brand New And Better Thought™, but rather to pause and acknowledge our current think-feel-act cycle exactly as it is.

Take a moment to do an Anchor Scan (page 183) or a Soothing Recall (page 191), imagining a loved one reading your Thought Work Protocol alongside you. Deciding to move forward with compassion, you're going to hold nonjudgmental space for your habitual thoughts, accepting that this is your current interpretation based in your history, while honoring that you learned to think this way for a reason. You are not broken. You are not stupid. You shouldn't have figured this out sooner. None of that, my love, *porfa y gracias*. Your inner children have been holding beliefs that kept you safe for decades. *You* have always been doing your best even if your mean inner-critic gremlin says otherwise (and come on—do you really wanna listen to that meanie-pants anyway?!). And, my sweetling, adult you has agency that kiddo you didn't have. You get to hold yourself lovingly accountable for your interpretations—recognizing that you came by them rightly, while also working to choose thoughts about yourself and your role in the world that bring positive results for your life that can ripple outward to have positive impacts on those you love, your community, and the world.

A big part of taking accountability is to name where our habitual interpretation might be coming from. Remember, our habitual thoughts are shaped by our experiences, perceptions, social location, and what we've paid attention to throughout our lives. What this means is that our personal histories, the legacies of our inner kiddos, our culture(s), and the broader presence of oppressive systems often show up in our interpretation line, and it's up to us to notice the voice of oppressive systems speaking through us—even and especially when we don't mean for it to.

For example, my client Eleanor had had it with her husband's lateness. A Black Jamaican-born man, Eithan joked often that he lived on "island time," but the habit of turning up thirty or forty minutes later than he said he would drove white, Massachusetts-born-and-raised Eleanor crazy. Every time he was even just five minutes late to their date night, or he "made her late" for a friend's party, she'd jump to criticizing. "I don't know why you're like this. 'Island time' isn't a thing, and even if it were, we don't live on an island, Eithan. We live in Boston. Why can't you just be on time for once? Don't you get that it's rude? You make me look bad with our friends!"

Eleanor came to our coaching sessions hurt and confused, holding tight to the story that Eithan just didn't care about her or her time. But what she didn't realize was the way she had unconsciously internalized a belief that punctuality is morally superior—a belief that is, in fact, deeply rooted in white Western colonial mandates. The interpretation Eleanor had of these situations—that she was being disrespected by her husband, that she didn't matter and wasn't "worth" being on time for—was rooted deeply in a belief that only one person's culture can be "right." Once Eleanor recognized where her interpretation came from, she saw that her feelings of disrespect were misplaced. She didn't want to cling to a belief that dismissed her husband's autonomy, reality, and dignity—especially when he was someone she loved deeply and who, in truth, treated her with great care and respect. As she loosened her grip on this story, she also realized how she had let his readiness to leave the house or not impact when *she* left. Leaving when she wanted, instead of waiting for him, was an option she hadn't even imagined before doing thought work. Three months after this call, Eleanor told me she had been hopping on the subway when she wanted to, letting Eithan take care of himself and his own departure, and they were both enjoying parties and events so much more when they each managed their own arrival. She stopped making his sense of time about her—no longer seeing his experience of time as a reflection of her worth or a personal slight, but simply as *his* way of moving through the world. Instead of trying to control his timeline, she let him manage his own arrival, freeing them both from unnecessary tension and allowing her to enjoy her own plans without resentment.

As you take accountability for your own interpretations, I invite you to look for ways that your thoughts have been colonized and informed by the expectations of oppressive systems like patriarchy, capitalism, and white-settler colonialism. Watch for statements wrapped up in all-or-nothing thinking, beliefs about "earning" or "deserving" love, care, or rest, and expectations around caregiving or caretaking. These systems can manifest in unexpected ways—like the internalized pressure to always "be productive" or "do more," rooted in capitalist ideals of extraction and exploitation. Every overfunctioner must question any thought in their own mind that whispers *lazy*—a word so often weaponized to keep us in cycles of overwork, self-sacrifice, and exhaustion, buffering against our feelings. Or the ways in which white-settler colonialism pushes ideas of rugged individualism, disconnecting us from communal care and shared responsibility, and prioritizing self-reliance at the expense of interdependence. Notice how thoughts create a moral hierarchy, where worth is attached to productivity, caregiving, or adherence to rigid standards. Even thoughts that seem relatively benign, like *I just need to tough it out* or *It's up to me to fix this,* reflect how these systems have taught us to devalue rest, softness, and community, prioritizing self-sacrifice and dominance over our own well-being. Recognizing these patterns is key to reclaiming your thoughts and allowing yourself the fullness of your humanity—beyond the confines of colonial expectations.

Again, my radiant star, this accountability does *not* mean that we are the sole inventor of all our thoughts! Those beliefs that you have to earn love or that rest is lazy and morally sus are stories we internalized to stay safe in the face of our family's expectations, and the pressures of patriarchal, white Western colonial, capitalist systems. Once we can see plainly that the interpretation we are operating from is not one we agree with or wish to perpetuate, we can choose a new thought to take its place.

Step 2: What Do I Want Instead?

In this step, we focus on the result(s) we'd like to see in our own lives. It is valid and understandable to want your daughter to want to spend time with you, or to wish that your partner could just do it right the first time, but we can only make choices for ourselves. We don't get to choose the thoughts, emotions, or actions of other people. We can only support ourselves to tell new stories, regulate our nervous systems, and behave in ways that affirm our worth and connection to others a little more each day.

For example, you could decide you want to create a result like one of the following:

I have time to start a new fitness routine and take care of myself.

I have more compassion for my partner (instead of focusing just on disappointments).

I can enjoy time talking with friends at my party (instead of playing hostess with the mostess).

I feel present to my own feelings when I receive feedback on my work.

I spend the day with my parent without yelling or feeling invalidated.

I respond honestly and do not just say, "I'm fine," when a friend asks.

Once you have a sense of what you would like your new result to be, write it down in your journal.

Step 3: Create a Bridge Thought

The most common mistake I see among my clients when they begin their intentional protocols is that they choose a new thought that is far too grand and aspirational and then beat themselves up when it's not achievable. Knowing as we do now that our thoughts create our feelings, which fuel our actions, it's tempting to say, "Amazing! I'll just tell myself that I'm the best and there's nothing to worry about, *et voilà!* Emotional Outsourcing be gone!"

My love, if only it were that simple.

Emotional bypassing and false positivity will not serve you, and glorifying the idea that a "positive" thought is a morally superior choice, or falling prey to our all-or-nothing perfectionist tendencies and overcorrecting to a #goodvibesonly mind-set is just another way of shutting ourselves out of our real, embodied experience. I've had clients try to front with "I'm happy my husband cheated if that's what he needed," face scrunched in hurt, a quiet tear rolling down their cheek, perpetuating the neural groove that their husband's needs and desires matter more than their own hurt—*ouch!* It's okay to be *wicked grumped* about things that are *not* okay—but it's vital that you don't gaslight yourself into pretending that something lousy is actually great. You cannot strong-arm yourself into believing some BS new result, my darling, and it's not loving or feminist to try to. So, instead, we're going to pick a thought that we can actually believe, right here, right now.

Specifically, we're going to choose a *bridge thought*—an intermediate interpretation that lets us *sneak up on our minds*, shifting our perspective *gently and gradually* rather than triggering alarm bells with forced positivity or overcorrection. Bridge thoughts use lots of adjectives and adverbs to introduce a new thought while simultaneously maintaining enough cognitive distance that the thought feels plausible to us. Here are some common phrases we can use to start bridge thoughts:

- I'm learning . . .
- It is possible . . .
- Self-love tells me that . . .
- Sometimes I can believe . . .
- My best friend believes . . .
- I'm starting to practice . . .
- I am open to . . .

You'll know you've found a bridge thought that serves you when you can say it out loud without cringing to the point of wanting to die, feeling flutters of panic in your body, or conjuring the sneering specter of your inner critic, eager to remind you that "that's kinda BS and we both know it." For example, the thought *I accept my mother and her codependent thought habits and I meet her with full love and radical acceptance* is so dreamy, right? But when your relationship with your mother is more thorns than roses, that thought can be hard to believe in a real way because, well, it's not real yet. So you might try on the bridge thought *I'm working to slowly accept my mother and her codependent habits, even if I can't meet her with radical acceptance right now.*

To get from the ouchy thought *I'm so friggin codependent; why can't I just be normal?!* you might try *I learned to have codependent habits as a kid as a survival skill and I am willing to entertain the possibility that at some point I might be able to take a small step toward knowing what I think and feel without having to check with someone else every time.* The more cushion, the merrier! I once had a client who wanted to leave her marriage, but was afraid of what her religious family would think, use the bridge thought *I'm learning that it is possible that sometimes I can believe that maybe my family might love me even if I leave my marriage.* It was a mouthful, but it worked! Give yourself space to be a human with a human mind and nervous system. I promise that slow and steady bridge thoughts are the only way you're going to rewire those neural grooves for the long haul, my lovely, *Because Science.*

Now, my overachieving darlings, I know it can be hard to believe that such a deliciously small, gentle step can impact your experience or ever help you to overcome those Emotional Outsourcing neural pathways. It takes a little faith, but those bridge thoughts can pack a surprising punch over time. Let's revisit April's situation to show you what I mean. You'll remember that her original protocol looked like this:

Observation (bare-bones, court-admissible facts, no adjectives or adverbs): *I asked my boyfriend to go to the art museum; he didn't say that he* ***wanted*** *to go, so instead, we went to a basketball game.*

Interpretation (reactions, automatic thoughts; what meaning am I making? what story am I telling? nervous system state): *I can't do what I want unless the other person is totally on board and it's up to me to ensure they're on board, and even though he didn't say he doesn't want to go to the museum, I don't want to risk him having a bad time and it being my fault. If he's not enthusiastic, I'll feel exposed, like I'm asking for too much, like I'm needy. If I push for what I want, I could be rejected or dismissed, and I'd rather abandon my own desires than feel that sting. Nervous system response: Dorsal vagal (collapsed, shut down, defeated).*

Feeling (emotion, then physical sensations): *resentment—hot cheeks, heavy limbs, fogginess, with tingling in my hands.*

Actions (what you did/didn't do): *I interpreted his lack of enthusiasm for my plan to mean he didn't want to do it; I projected my fears that I don't matter onto him; from my people-pleasing habits I decided to do what I felt he wanted more than what I wanted even though he didn't say no to my plan: Agreed to go to the game despite wanting to go to the museum; smiled and acted like it wasn't a big deal; minimized my own feelings; ruminated afterward about how they never do what I want; avoided bringing up my disappointment later.*

Result (what was the outcome of those actions in *your* life?): *I declined to go to the art museum because my boyfriend said words. I prioritized my boyfriend's interests over my own, reinforced the belief that my interests never matter, felt more distant from myself and him, reinforced a dorsal response, missed an opportunity to advocate for myself, created distance with myself.*

When we sat down to create an intentional protocol together, April told me that what she really wanted was to feel like her interests matter and are respected. She took accountability for not believing that her interests mattered enough to be worth advocating for and recognized that this habitual interpretation likely started in childhood when her whole world was ruled by her older, sportier sibling's baseball schedule. What she wanted to do on the weekend was rarely more important than the big game.

Moreover, April recognized that this pattern of deference to her partner's desires is rooted in the patriarchal conditioning that women should be submissive, passive, and accommodating. She also saw that she wasn't just prioritizing his interests—she was avoiding vulnerability. The moment he wasn't explicitly excited about her idea, she felt exposed, like asking for what she wanted was risky. She assumed that if he wasn't immediately elated, pushing for the museum would mean forcing him, making her a burden. It felt safer to preemptively abandon her desire than to risk rejection or conflict.

While she cares about her boyfriend, she no longer wanted to prioritize his interests over her own, but jumping all the way to "I matter just as much as you!" was too much (she noticed how her body got tense and sweaty just imagining what it would be like to believe that, much less say it out loud, a sign of some sympathetic activation). Instead, we came to the bridge thought *Sometimes I can believe that my interests might just matter too.*

The next week, she found herself in a similar situation: She wanted her boyfriend to come with her to a barbecue with her friends, but he wanted to go see the new Marvel movie together. Instead of defaulting to the interpretation "My interests don't matter," she pulled out her bridge thought. Instead of going numb and agreeing out of habit, April was able to stay more present to herself. She noticed the familiar tug to fold, to shrink back, but this time, she paused. From that more grounded place, she told her boyfriend that he got to pick last time, and it was important to her that he get to know her friends better. Her stomach clenched for a second, waiting for pushback, but it never came. That tiny shift in her thought derailed her habitual cycle and allowed her to move into a more ventral vagal state—connected, clear, and able to advocate for herself. She felt steadier, more solid in her own skin, proof that she could hold on to herself and stay in connection at the same time. She was able to take a different action to honor her dignity and her desires just because it mattered to her.

Pretty incredible stuff, huh?

Kitten Step: What If It's Not a Problem?

If you're struggling to find a bridge thought that works for you (or, *ahem*, you're ruminating and overthinking it), try one of my favorites on for size: "…and it's not a problem." When we're deep in Emotional Outsourcing, our nervous system scans for problems constantly. Not because we're dramatic or nitpicky, but because we've been conditioned to see discomfort as danger. If something is *off*, our brains leap into action: Fix it! Solve it! Control it! That cluttered countertop? A personal failing. That weird look from your friend? A sign of imminent rejection. Someone else's body being bigger than you think bodies *should* be—or someone having tattoos or piercings? Proof that they're doing something wrong—and that you need to comment on it, lest anyone think you approve of how other people choose to live in and care for their own bodies…which might mean something bad about *you*. That guy taking "too long" to order coffee? A violation of an unspoken social contract that *must* mean something. We become hypervigilant, disconnected from presence, and convinced that every irritation, mistake, or difference is a crisis.

Why? Because our shame has taught us that if there's a problem, we must be the problem. And if we're the problem, we have to *fix* it—fast. So we criticize, overfunction, ruminate, fawn—anything to neutralize the perceived threat before it confirms our worst fear: that we are fundamentally unlovable.

And so, my love, we ask:

- What if it's not a problem?
- What if your toddler's aversion to broccoli isn't a problem?
- What if your mother-in-law's penchant for hideous sweaters isn't a problem?

- What if the guy taking "too long" to order coffee isn't a problem?

Tacking on "*...and it's not a problem*" to our interpretation can interrupt the cycle—it takes the nervous system out of threat mode and turns down the heat on the story we're telling ourselves. And when the intensity cools, there's more space for new thoughts, different feelings, and fresh choices.

~~~

My brave bean, as hard as it can be to get honest with ourselves about the role we play in creating outcomes in our own lives—and specifically how often the thoughts we entertain cause us pain and keep us stuck—there is such liberation in knowing that you do *not* have to agree with those old stories. When you change your thoughts, you recalibrate your entire experience of life. You will undoubtedly still confront the challenges that come from being humans in the world. Life will be lifey. Your car won't start. Dinner will burn. A package won't arrive. You'll forget someone's birthday. But you don't have to stay stuck in the neural groove that tells you those situations mean anything about you as a perfect human animal.

Engaging daily with the Thought Work Protocol as you continue to widen your window of capacity with the somatic practices you learned in chapter 6 will give you more and more space to *choose* how you want to think, feel, or act (or not act) in any given moment. Lovingly, slowly, you get to decline to think in ways that no longer serve you. Each time you create space to pause, to compassionately own the role that you play in your think-feel-act cycle, and choose a bridge thought over your habitual interpretation, you take one more step to reinforce the knowledge that you are good, whole, worthy, safe, and loved.
~~~

JOURNAL PROMPTS
NOTICING THE BIG PICTURE

The specifics of each situation you encounter in your life may vary widely, but it's also true that we who wade in ye olde Emotional Outsourcing waters are creatures of habit. Pausing to notice broader themes in our think-feel-act cycles builds self-awareness, which helps us spot our thought errors quicker each time. As you get the hang of the Thought Work Protocol and creating bridge thoughts, spend some time reflecting on these common scenarios:

1. Reflect on a time when you felt "stuck." What thoughts and feelings contributed to that sense of being trapped, and how did they impact your actions? What was really going on, factually, in the moment, and how did you habitually interpret that experience? What's a different, less stuck-making interpretation?

2. Write about a feeling you tend to avoid. How do your thoughts about that feeling shape your actions when it shows up? For example, I avoid feeling vulnerable around others, and that avoidance makes me withdraw or overcompensate, which creates distance and prevents genuine connection.

3. Think of a situation where you overcommitted or agreed to something you didn't want to do. What was your interpretation of the moment that led to that choice? What were you making it mean about you if you did that thing or not?

....

....

....

4. Consider a recent interaction where you felt dismissed or overlooked. What thoughts did you have about yourself in that moment, and what might a bridge thought sound like here?

....

....

....

5. Reflect on a time when you compared yourself to others. What assumptions did you make, and how did those thoughts impact your feelings and actions?

....

....

....

6. Describe a moment when you felt disconnected from your needs. What thoughts might have pulled you away from noticing or meeting your own needs?

....

....

....

7. Write about a situation where you held back from speaking up. What thoughts kept you silent, and how did that impact your relationship with yourself?

8. Think about a time when you acted in a way you later regretted. What thought-feeling-action sequence led you there, what state was your nervous system in, and what might have shifted the outcome?

9. April, the woman in our example, projected her fear that her desires don't matter onto her boyfriend, thus keeping herself from doing what she wants while telling the story that it was about him not prioritizing her—is that a pattern or habit of yours? What might you want to do instead?

Chapter 8

Boundaries, Limits, and Direct Communication

If I polled my clients about whether they would rather sit in the freezing rain for an hour without an umbrella or set a boundary, especially with a parent or partner, I think a solid 90 percent would pick pneumonia. Because our sense of self, safety, belonging, and worthiness is so tied up in others' opinions about us, it's existentially terrifying to set limits, say no, draw a boundary and stick to it, and pretty much do anything that might upset the proverbial apple cart of their positive regard for us—even when it makes us feel unheard, unseen, taken advantage of and disrespected, we prefer that comfortable hell to the unknown risk of speaking up for ourselves.

And so we stay spinning in our Emotional Outsourcing habits because it's pretty darn challenging to maintain an embodied sense of self when you're constantly saying yes when you mean no, resenting the people you love for not reading your mind and knowing your limits, which you haven't communicated, while doing your very best to ignore your needs in relationships because you're so scared to lose the people you're scared to be honest with. Quite the doozy, that one.

Turns out, people can't just read your mind to know what you need—*lousy news* for those of us still holding out hope that our partner will magically intuit it without us having to say a word. So in this chapter, we're going to learn how to put the self-awareness, self-support, and agency we've been fostering into practice as we acquaint ourselves with our limits, practice direct communication, and learn to set and enforce our boundaries when needed.

While you might be tempted to throw this book clear across the room—and I get that impulse—I want to teach you all of this because my life got so much better when I learned how to speak my mind clearly and directly. Healthy, loving communication starts with being able to trust yourself to know what's right for you and to speak up for it, and it is a cornerstone of relationships based in mutual respect, autonomy, and emotional safety. Every time we recognize and assert our needs, we steer away from icky people-pleasing and codependent dynamics and toward more self-respect and interdependence in our relationships. My love, I know you didn't do all this work on yourself only to accept relationships that pinch, that hurt, and that don't allow you to respect yourself. In my experience, life is way more fulfilling when you're actually getting what you want, and even better when you can do that in community with others.

LIMITS AND BOUNDARIES: WHERE I START AND YOU END

The term "boundaries" gets thrown around a *lot* these days. The internet would have you believe that boundaries are onetime limits that we set about other people's behavior, effectively you saying, "Ewww, David! Don't do that!" but that's not quite how it works, my darlings, so let's slow down and take it from the top.

I like to think about boundaries as the invisible line between two neighbors' yards. That property line is where your sovereignty ends and where your neighbor's domain begins. You do not get to tell them what they can or can't plant in their garden, and by the same token, they don't get to tell you what you can plant in yours. (Of course, this is all very different if you live in a neighborhood with an HOA, which in this metaphor embodies the spirit of the oppressive patriarchal, capitalist, white-settler colonial systems that limit what *everyone* can have in their garden and punish those who do not follow the rules, but I digress.)

Most days, we don't need to spend a lot of time communicating about the property line. It's there, we keep our side of the street clean, end of story. But let's say your neighbor gets a dog. If they want to let Oscar poop in their front lawn, that's up to them. If, however, Oscar makes a habit of coming into *your* yard to do his business, well, then they're crossing a line, and it's time to start communicating.

Before we even get to boundaries, we first have to recognize our limits. A limit is the internal line we recognize within ourselves—what we can tolerate, what feels safe or aligned, and what we're simply *not* available for. Limits are personal, internal, and self-honoring, guiding our choices and shaping how we respond to situations. Unlike boundaries, which are about how we act in response to others, limits are what we hold within ourselves to protect our energy, well-being, and values. For example, let's say you know that you can't stand the smell of cigarette smoke—it makes you feel sick and gives you a headache. That's a limit—your body's boundary with the world. But how you respond to that limit is where boundaries come in.

While limits are internal knowing, boundaries are how we communicate and uphold those limits in the world. Limits help us recognize what does and doesn't work for us; boundaries are the action we take to protect those limits. A boundary is a clear statement about what we will do to take care of ourselves if someone or something crosses over into our yard without permission. Boundaries mark what we're okay with and what we're not, separating our needs and values from the expectations and demands of the world around us.

While we form boundaries in response to other people, they are only ever about us and our own behavior. For that reason, we always state boundaries as "If you do X, I will do Y." For example, if your limit is that cigarette smoke makes you sick, your boundary might be: *If you smoke near me, I will move to another space.* If your limit is that yelling feels overwhelming and shuts you down, your boundary might be: *If you raise your voice at me, I will step away from the conversation until we can talk calmly.*

For example:

- If you raise your voice, I'm going to leave the conversation.
- If you are more than ten minutes late to our appointment, we'll have to reschedule.
- I have a chronic illness, and if you continue not to mask around me, I'm not going to spend time with you anymore.
- If you come into the room while I'm meditating, I'm going to ask you to leave until I've finished.
- If you keep telling other people the things I've told you in confidence, I'm going to scale back on what I share with you.

Boundaries are *always* in the first person, are *always* focused on our own actions, and are about *you* taking care of *you*. The goal of a boundary is not to change someone else's behavior or to make decisions for them. I'll say it again, love, because it is super-duper important: Your boundaries are not about anyone except you. They're a reflection of how you choose to care for yourself when someone else's actions, needs, or priorities conflict with your own.

It's a statement that "I need X to feel safe (or respected or whatever), and if that doesn't happen, I will take Y action to take care of myself."

Boundaries versus Ultimatums

Whereas boundaries are calm, flexible statements about how we will care for ourselves, ultimatums are rigid threats that are intended to control another person's behavior—to compel someone to act how you want them to. "Marry me or I'll break up with you" is a classic; other familiar ones include "Give me a raise or I'll quit," "If you don't attend the family gathering, I'll never speak to you again," and "If you don't give me your full attention exactly when I need it and exactly the way I want, I will shut down and won't be vulnerable with you again." While these statements follow our same "if/then" framework, and while some of the underlying needs and limits may be the same, boundaries are never about manipulating, threatening, or coercing another person. Boundaries are about honoring your needs *without* violating someone else's autonomy.

The easiest way to tell if you're setting a boundary or issuing an ultimatum is to check in on your nervous system. If you're activated—you notice urgency, anger, anxiety, or a need to defend yourself—it's likely an ultimatum. Boundaries are something we set from our calm, social ventral vagal state, where we're grounded in ourselves and our self-worth. Boundaries aren't about trying to make anyone feel anything or proving anything to anyone, and are def not used to punish others—they're about you taking care of yourself. When you set a boundary, you're not bracing for a fight or trying to avoid one—you're simply expressing what you need to maintain your emotional and physical equilibrium.

WHY WE DON'T SET BOUNDARIES

It's so common for my clients to feel bad about themselves for not being a boundaries superstar from the jump, and I want to normalize how challenging knowing and expressing our limits can be for us Emotional Outsourcing cuties. Our young minds and nervous systems often learned that boundaries were not allowed, for the rather straightforward reason that having boundaries requires developing a strong sense of self. To know where I end and you begin, I have to have an embodied sense of self—and, my darling, that's not something that our codependent, people-pleasing habits allow us to do. Especially when we grow up with enmeshment or parentification woven into our family blueprints, our sense of whose yard is whose—and whether we even *get* to say something when the neighbor starts taking tomatoes from our garden—gets real fuzzy, real fast. Without role models for healthy boundary setting, it either doesn't cross our minds to set them or we have absolutely no idea where to start. Many of us grew up in environments where boundaries were ignored, bulldozed, or outright framed as selfish, leaving adult-us feeling guilty, hesitant, and unsure about setting them now. Our deep-seated desire for approval, acceptance, and love can fully overshadow our ability to prioritize our own well-being and establish healthy limits. As long as we're looking outside ourselves for safety, worth, and connection, telling someone to kindly get off our metaphorical lawn (and keep their mitts off the tomatoes!) is going to feel wicked challenging—maybe even impossible.

As a result, there's often a disconnect between what we want to do, what we feel, and what we actually do. For example, let's say your friend invited you to a party and you feel an immediate "ugh" in your shoulders. There are always so many people you don't know and the last time you went to one of her parties you were zapped for a week. But instead of texting back, "Shoot, I can't make it, but thanks for including me!" you say, "Of course! See you there! What can I bring?!" and are full of regret the moment the text whooshes away through the ether. So you go, expensive bottle of wine in hand, because you said you would, and you don't want her to be disappointed or mad, to think less of you or judge you. You stand there and make small talk and hate being there the whole time, building resentment toward yourself and eroding any trust that you can make good choices for you—feeling disappointed in and mad at yourself, thinking less of you and judging you...

When we don't set boundaries, we keep ourselves stuck in obligation, undermine our needs and relationships, overstep our windows of capacity on the regular, and reinforce our habitual think-feel-act cycles. I can do my utmost to believe that my needs matter, but if I consistently schedule over my alone time, or put off that doctor's appointment because work feels more important, or let my parent ignore my requests, well... the self-abandonment cycle prevails.

By contrast, healthy boundaries protect our dignity and autonomy. They act as clear statements about who we are, what we value, what is acceptable to us, and how we choose to navigate our space in the world, without trying to change anyone else and what they're up to. Even, and perhaps especially, when others aren't willing or able to honor them, our boundaries show our commitment to showing up for ourselves, rather than conform to others' expectations and demands at our expense.

NO, BOUNDARIES AREN'T SELFISH—THEY'RE RESENTMENT PREVENTION

The chief fear I hear from my clients is that boundaries are selfish—closely followed by "But what if they don't like my boundary?" and "But what if they leave?" My love, let's pause: Whose story is that? Who told you that honoring yourself—living with respect for the needs and preferences that make you *you* and keep you well—is selfish? I think we can all agree that it was not your realest self, my perfect marigold.

I know I point a finger at the patriarchy whenever I hear this (maybe a middle finger? who's to say?), because it teaches women that our value comes from the support we offer to others; we are taught to be a constant endless resource to the men around us, rather than people deserving resources of our own. I mean, women get called selfish for taking care of ourselves, where men get called, well . . . nothing. It's just what they do, and no one has anything to say about it. I want to state this plainly: Asserting your boundaries isn't causing trouble or being a nuisance, even if the system is doing its best to make you believe that. When you set a boundary, that is you doing your best to take care of yourself, affirm your value, and advocate for relationships that feel nurturing and safe.

In fact, boundaries are mandatory for interdependence and community care. When we're aware of where we end and where others begin, it creates space for consent, respect, and mutuality. Communicating regularly about our own needs, wants, and limits helps us to respect the needs, wants, and limits of others, and that mutual understanding builds trust. Remember, my love, that in this family, boundaries are not impenetrable brick walls. We set boundaries because we *want* to connect—and we value ourselves enough to do so in ways that maintain our autonomy and dignity. A healthy boundary is dynamic, adaptable, and subject to our discretion. Boundaries are not fixed structures; rather, they can shift, evolve, or even be completely removed as our needs and circumstances change.

Setting a boundary doesn't require you to be mean, aggressive, or harsh, and you don't have to hurt any feelings—not at all! It's about owning your choices and preferences, clearly stating what flies with you and what doesn't, and how you're going to handle it. Clear communication about our needs and boundaries is a kindness, my love. Don't believe me? Which situation would you prefer: starting a job where your new boss says, "Do whatever you want! We're pretty chill around here," only to find out later that you've gone against protocol (surprise! there's a protocol after all!), or getting sent a PDF that spells out exactly the way the company handles situations? Most people would choose the clear guidance. When we fail to be explicit about our boundaries, we doom our relationships to resentment and miscommunication, ensuring that our needs aren't met and that the people around us can't respect our limits even if they want to. You, and the people you love, deserve more than that.

Boundaries and Privilege

Darling, I want to get real with you: Enforcing a boundary can be a privilege. While we are always free to know our limits and do our best to honor them by communicating our needs, it is also true that for a variety of reasons it is not always safe or possible to uphold our boundaries the way we would like to.

There is enormous privilege in being able to set boundaries with family members, particularly in situations where cultural norms, financial dependence, physical safety, or childcare needs are at issue. Gender norms are quick to punish women who do not give away their time, resources, and energy in service of others. Economic pressures and class disparities create power imbalances that make it harder for folks with fewer resources to assert their needs. And the realities of late-stage capitalism and the lack of a social safety net for U.S. workers can make boundaries around work-life balance somewhere between challenging and impossible.

What I want to challenge you to consider is whether the consequences of setting a boundary are guaranteed, or if they're projections and worries. When a boundary like "Hey, the next time you assign me a project without asking, I'm going to say no" or "I'm not available for that outside of work hours, but I can address it on Monday," carries the very real consequence of getting you fired, or subtler, more malicious consequences like getting you labeled "difficult to work with" and blacklisted, my dove, your mind-body may be absolutely correct that boundaries are not safe in that case. You deserve to have a say in what takes up your mental and emotional space, time, resources, and energy, my love. If a capital-*B* boundary isn't possible for you right now, give yourself grace, and do your best to honor your needs, capacity, and self in the ways that you can (and if you DO set a boundary, make sure to CC HR on that email).

KNOW YOUR LIMITS

The process of setting and enforcing boundaries starts with knowing your limits. We've all felt that energy inside that lets us know that whatever is happening needs to pause, shift, or change. A limit is that threshold at which our bodies tell us, "*Basta*—enough—done." More scientifically, it's the point at which a person feels discomfort, stress, or challenged, or feels unwilling or unable to cope with a particular situation.[1] Not all people's limits are the same, and they aren't static either. Our limits will vary based on our emotions, values, past experiences, body, age, mental health, trauma history, mental load, level of extroversion, neurobiology—all the way down to how much water we've had recently, or whether it's especially hot or cold outside.

You might think of limits as personal, invisible markers that help us gauge our comfort and capacity and determine when to pump the brakes. The felt experience of a limit can manifest as discomfort, anxiety, or frustration, or perhaps it's a simple "I'm done" with little emotion or a sense of overwhelm. Limits let us know when we need to take action to support or protect our well-being or regain a sense of control, so we can pause, step back, say no, or make adjustments in our life to avoid pushing ourselves beyond what we can comfortably handle.

I used to have no idea when enough was enough and would push myself way past my limit at work, in the gym, when studying. I was deep in my Emotional Outsourcing, and like all of us folks who have walked the codependent, perfectionist, people-pleasing tightrope, I was keen to believe that the limit did not exist. When we live from Emotional Outsourcing, we've blown past our limits and borrowed energy from tomorrow so often that we have an unrealistic sense of our emotional and mental capacities. In relationships with others, we have not felt safe to say no or to ask others to accommodate our needs, so we do everything beyond our capacity to keep the people around us good, because when they're good, we're good too. It's a recipe for burnout, resentment, and even more self-abandonment—precisely the opposite of what we're trying to learn, my loves.

We get in touch with our limits by noticing, first and foremost, our nervous system state. Our limits are the metaphorical frame of our window of capacity—when we live with respect for our capacity, we're hanging out in ventral vagal. When we get dysregulated, slipping into sympathetic activation, dorsal, or hanging out in functional freeze, it's a sure sign that we're outside our limits for the moment. Taking time daily to map our bodily sensations and emotions to understand our nervous system state will tell you a *lot* about whether you've reached (or surpassed) your limit. You'll also have limits that map to your core values (e.g., honesty, family, community, autonomy, spirituality), as well as your specific needs around things like personal space, communication, time, emotions, and solitude.

I recommend that you get as specific as possible about what matters to you and what sets you up to feel best. The clearer you are for yourself, the better you'll be able to recognize when someone or something is trespassing on your limits and (eventually) communicate about those boundaries. For example, my client

Rebecca has learned over the years that she can handle pretty much anything so long as she gets morning movement and time each day to enjoy fictional content. The form those take can vary: Some days she can train for that half-marathon and others it's just a quick sun salutation; an audiobook might sub in when she doesn't have time for an episode of that new TV show. Whatever may be happening, Rebecca knows that when those two core needs aren't being met, she's living beyond her limits and it's time to evaluate whether that new client *really* needs a 7 a.m. meeting, or whether the coffee ritual her husband loves is really allowing her to be her favorite self.

Ultimately, enough is a decision, not an amount, my love—because only you get to define what's enough for you. You get to draw lines in the sand wherever you need to safeguard your mental, emotional, physical, social, and spiritual health, knowing that you can redraw them at any point should you wish to.

Kitten Step: Red Flag Feelings

Limits can start to sound very intellectual when we describe them, but they're first and foremost felt sensations. Emotions like anger, resentment, guilt, irritability, or annoyance; feeling taken advantage of, disrespected, or run down; and physical symptoms like chronic pain, GI distress, migraine, or fatigue are all red flags that you may be exceeding your limits. As you get familiar with your real capacity in a given moment, I encourage you to notice when those emotions and sensations show up most often—and to explore them through thought work. It may be that your current action isn't serving you, and that it's time to choose a boundary instead.

START WITH AN INTERNAL BOUNDARY

So, now that you're starting to notice what you're up for and what pushes you over the edge, the next step is to call everyone you know and tell them in no uncertain terms that you're no longer available for anything that pushes your limits . . . right? Nope! Not even a little bit.

One of the greatest misconceptions about boundaries is that they have to be externalized and overcommunicated to "count," and that's just not true, my dove. Our boundaries are about our own actions, and the first step is actually to communicate with *ourselves* about how we'd like to handle a given situation. We do this by setting an internal boundary based on our limits. It follows the same "If they do X, I'm going to do Y" formula, but is often something you can enact without having a big conversation. For example, let's say you have a limit about being around intoxicated people. Once someone starts slurring their words, or hits whatever level of inebriation makes you say, "I'm out!" you can make a quiet, self-loving exit. No need for an excuse or explanation—you can just leave. An internal boundary in other situations might sound like:

Limit: I need eight hours of sleep to function well.

Internal boundary: My phone goes on airplane mode at 9 p.m., and I won't check or respond to messages until morning.

Limit: I have a low tolerance for last-minute changes to my schedule.

Internal boundary: When someone asks for a meeting with less than twenty-four hours' notice, I will decline and offer a time to meet that works better for me.

Limit: I'm fasting for Ramadan and won't eat until after sundown.

Internal boundary: I'll go to my friend's birthday party, but I'll tell her I can't be there until eight so that I can honor my fast with ease and without stress.

Limit: I need at least thirty minutes to myself in the morning or I get overwhelmed.

Internal boundary: On our family vacation, I will get up early to go for a solo walk and have coffee by myself before I join the group for the day.

Notice how none of those boundaries requires you to explain your limit to someone else before you take care of you the way you want to? You get to move from *knowing* your limit to *honoring* it, on your terms. Internal boundaries are not passive-aggressive, isolating or avoidant ways of dealing with challenging situations, nor are they a tool for manipulation. They're the first line of honoring our own needs and capacity. And, of course, not every situation can be resolved with an internal boundary alone. When that's the case, it's time for the next step: direct communication.

COMMUNICATE DIRECTLY

One of the trickiest habits we learn in Emotional Outsourcing homes is to communicate in ways that guard against conflict or abandonment, better known as passive aggression. In Spanish, when someone says something opaque, passive-aggressive, or generally not clear and honest, we call it *un indirecta*—an indirect. When someone says, "Yeah, that's fine, wherever you want to go for lunch—I'm good with whatever" instead of "I'm vegetarian so I'd rather not go to a barbecue spot," they are being indirect instead of being honest. When a parent said, "Oh, is that what you're wearing?" instead of "Hey! I love the color but I don't think that's appropriate for our activity today," their passive aggression undermined your choice and your self-trust that you can make good decisions without their input.

Folks with Emotional Outsourcing habits are masters of *indirectas*. We skirt the issue with passive-aggressive language—sigh, and say, "Don't worry, it's fine," when it's anything but. This tendency to be unclear in our speech, to project our fears, and to read into what others are saying (in case they're doing the same thing we are) comes from the stories we learned in childhood that people won't like what we say, think, or have to offer if we're honest, and we better not upset anyone! As a result, clear communication feels really risky to us. Speaking up might make you a burden, show exactly how you're too much, and risk you being rejected, abandoned, critiqued, ostracized. Displeasing or disappointing others feels as smart as drinking lava, so we opt for hinting, sighing, eye rolling, passive-aggressive comments, or just hoping someone will read our minds rather than being straightforward.

At its core, direct communication is the difference between deflecting with "Oh, I'm fine" and clearly stating "No, thank you" or "Yes, please" when someone offers you a glass of water. In direct communication we prioritize transparency, trust, and respect. That requires vulnerability, but the courage to express ourselves openly creates the foundation for healthier and more fulfilling interactions. We know we're communicating directly when we express ourselves honestly and authentically, without filtering ourselves through fear of judgment or rejection.

Direct communication is *not*, as some seem to believe, an excuse to say whatever's on your mind without regard for the other person and justify it in the name of "just being honest." For example, sharing a process thought (remember those from the Thought Work Protocol?) and following all of that up with, "What? I'm just being direct!" is *not* direct communication. That's dumping a bunch of your thoughts and opinions on someone else, and it certainly didn't communicate what *you* needed.

Lemme say this again: You are allowed to ask for exactly what you want, and if you want communication to happen a certain way or conflict handled a certain way, then you have to state it clearly. Don't make it weird; just make the request. Do you want flowers on Fridays? Ask for them. Want to be in charge of this account but not that one? Gotta tell 'em. Because, my love, yes. You do have to communicate your needs and wants out loud to other people.

But here's the kicker: Making a request doesn't mean you're owed a yes. You get to ask for anything you want, and the people in your life get to say no. The problem comes when we expect a yes and get mad if we don't get it—when a request turns into a demand or an expectation, and we hold it against someone for having their own preferences, limits, or capacity. Asking for what you want isn't about control; it's about clarity. And just as you have the right to ask, they have the right to answer in a way that reflects their own needs.

Staying wed to the story that it "doesn't count" unless they read your mind is a misdirected protective mechanism. "If we don't ask," our fearful inner children whisper, "then the other person can't say no, and if they say no that means we don't matter, and if we don't matter, we're not safe . . ." and that particular ignorance feels quite blissful. So, in an attempt to guard your tender underbelly, to keep you from getting too vulnerable or exposing your true self, you decline to say, "I matter, and this is what I want." But the truth is, real, reciprocal connection requires that we risk both yes and no.

More importantly, nobody can cross a limit that they don't know about. All those years of deferring to others, hiding or chameleoning your needs, and keeping everyone around you happy as clams has taught them that you are a limitless wonder woman, available for anything and everything, impervious to silly mortal obstacles like needs. Any attempt on their part to check in on you is likely met with, "Oh no, I'm totally fine! For sure! It's no problem, honest!" and, my little buttercup, that ends here and now!

There is no need to shame ourselves for behaving this way and keeping ourselves safe the best way we knew how, and it's time to see how much that habit hurts us and those we love. It's unkind and unfair to both people in a relationship for us to hope that they'll intuit our limits and for us to resent them for not mind reading.

Once we realize what our internal boundaries are, and especially if we notice one has been crossed, our first step is to try directly communicating about it. Sometimes a quick "Hey, I don't love when you call me that, could you stop, please?" or "I really need some alone time right now" can be enough. How you choose to communicate is up to you, though most often we have two options: Share what you're feeling or make a request. Let's see how both might work for you.

Option 1: Share What You're Wanting, Needing, or Feeling

My client Gina was struggling in her relationship with her friend Maya, who had a tendency to make decisions for the group without asking anyone. It wasn't malicious—Maya was an eldest daughter who loved to take charge and had her own fair share of perfectionist habits to combat—but whenever they tried to plan something together, Gina felt taken for granted and disrespected. Things really came to a head one day as they sat in a coffee shop, Maya rambling on about the *cutest* house she'd picked for a group trip, telling Gina how much she owed her... when Gina hadn't even been asked if she wanted to go, or if that weekend worked for her. She noticed the lump in her throat, the frustration, and Gina's thoughts grew louder: *I don't want to feel this way every time we make plans. I deserve to be part of the conversation.*

Palms sweating, Gina decided that today was the day she was going to speak up. "Hey, Maya, I appreciate all the thought you've put into this, but can I talk to you about something? I've been feeling a little left out when it comes to plans. Like, with this trip—no one asked if I even wanted to go. I'm not saying it was intentional, but it's been happening a lot lately, and it hurts." Gina wasn't really sure how Maya would respond, but she surprised her by reacting with immediate concern. "Oh my god, Gina, I'm so sorry! I didn't mean to, but you're right, I never even asked you. I've just been assuming that you're cool with whatever. I'm really sorry—I should've asked, and I'm really glad you told me how you were feeling. I'll do better to include you in plans, okay?"

A lifetime of codependent habits can make it challenging to remember that other people are adults too. Especially if parentification was part of your upbringing, your inner kiddos may still be holding on to the story that the adults around you can't be trusted to actually *be* adults without your support. But sometimes it really is enough just to express what we're feeling—exactly like Gina did in sharing her hurt with Maya. When people know the impact they're having on you, they're often more than willing to adjust their behavior as a result.

Kitten Step: Start with "Safer" People

Teaching your nervous system that it is safe enough to express your needs and wants is vital if you want to build your direct communication muscles. What that means, my love, is that you do *not* start directly communicating by telling your boomer parent all the ways they failed you. Instead, look for someone you already feel safe around or someone in a helping profession—maybe a friend who's a teacher, nurse, therapist, minister, or hairdresser. Let them know what you're working on, and get their consent to practice with them. Having someone listen actively and empathetically to your experience teaches your nervous system that you are safe, that your needs are not inherently scary to other people, and that you are still loved and accompanied when you express your true feelings.

Now, *mi amor,* commenting, "Wow! I'm so hungry!" hoping someone, anyone, else will start cooking dinner, is *not* the kind of sharing we're talking about here. Voicing your need as a hint or a Hail Mary that someone will snap into action the way you have trained yourself to do lives firmly in the land of *indirectas* and will not get you what you need. In these situations, we need to try a different tactic and make a request.

Option 2: Make a Request

Requests are how we tell others about our needs, wants, or preferences. They're an important part of asserting ourselves and collaborating effectively in relationships.[2] Something as simple as "Pass the salt please" or "Could you please slip your shoes off before coming inside? Thanks!" can help you clarify your needs and limits with others in real time and makes a world of difference to your experience in a relationship. Requests can range from simple, everyday things like asking for help with a task, to more significant and profound needs, such as requesting emotional support during challenging times. Regardless of the scope, each request carries with it an opportunity for deepening connection and understanding between folks who want to hear each other. My love, I want you to hear that last piece extra loud: Making a request isn't pushy, needy, weak, or codependent. Making a clear ask of another person offers them an opportunity to show up for you and to show you that they care. As it turns out, when you ask someone who cares about you to do something or to not do something because you prefer it that way, it's actually a gift to them.

Requests do require a certain amount of vulnerability—and that can be a daunting prospect for brains that are vigilant to any potential for rejection, abandonment, or confrontation. Making a request exposes us to the possibility of not having our needs met, which can be a significant source of anxiety and stress. Even so, learning to make requests effectively is a powerful step toward self-empowerment and healthier relationships.[3] When we acknowledge our needs and communicate them respectfully to others, we not only take responsibility for our own well-being but also open the door to more authentic and supportive interactions with those around us.

So many of my clients come to me frustrated about a lack of mutuality in one or more of their relationships. Sometimes that imbalance is due to the other person's underfunctioning or unwillingness to engage—which is absolutely real—but just as often, I see my clients unknowingly blocking opportunities for others to show up for them, even when they want to. If you're upset that your roommate literally never cleans the bathroom, have you tried asking them if they'd please do it this week? If you wish that another parent would take charge of the carpool every once in a while, have you tried texting the group to request that someone take Tuesday morning off your plate (so that you can finally be on time to yoga for once!)? So often we complain that no one is helping us, yet we don't look for alternatives to the plan we're drowning in, and when someone offers suggestions or help, we poo-poo them without giving them a fair shake—convinced it couldn't work because we're so mired in all the things that aren't working.

If we return to Gina's conversation with Maya, she could have equally tried making a request. For example, "Hey, Maya, thanks for all the thought you've been putting into this trip. I'm feeling frustrated because I wasn't actually asked if I even wanted to go. Next time we plan a group trip, can you please ask me first?"

Kitten Step: Pass the Salt?

Most of my clients would rather suffer an underseasoned chicken breast or reach awkwardly across the table than interrupt someone to ask them to pass the salt. We're so used to being on call for everyone else without asking for help in return that sometimes, frankly, we forget that other people are there to help us too. As you work up to making bigger requests, I want you to practice by making small, low-stakes requests of others. See if you can find one opportunity this week to ask something like:

- Hey, can I borrow a pen?
- Could you bring me a glass of water while you're up?
- Would you mind grabbing my charger while you're upstairs?
- Could you hand me a napkin please? Thanks!
- Can you turn out that light, please?

Notice how it feels in your body and, if you so choose, do a little thought work around what happened when you made that one small request. How did you feel? What result did it create for you? The more natural it feels to see the people around you as supports and resources, the more interdependence you can begin to source in those relationships.

People who have your best interests at heart want to do helpful things, they want to be caring for you, and they want to avoid doing things that upset you. If you are in a relationship where that is not true, I would encourage you to get curious about why you're staying in that relationship. I was there for a long time in my painful first marriage, and I've seen hundreds of clients stall out in their own romantic relationships, careers, and friendships, and I gotta tell you: In my personal and professional experience, if you've been making simple requests like these and the person in question doesn't seem to give an eff, chances are they won't ever change, so make your choices accordingly, my angel. The relationships that once felt "right" to our Emotional Outsourcing habits may no longer fit when we stop prioritizing the *existence* of a relationship over our *own* well-being and self-worth. Interdependence takes at least two, whether in friendship or partnership, and you deserve a community—and a partner—who steps up just as willingly and wholeheartedly as you do.

SET AN EXTERNAL BOUNDARY

Communicating our boundaries to others is often the first thing that comes to mind when we talk about boundaries, and for many of my clients, it feels overwhelming. As if direct communication weren't hard enough, the idea of telling someone what you're going to do in response to their behavior—especially when you *know* they may not like it—can be downright terrifying.

Take my client Dahlia, for example. She was burning the candle at both ends at her job, constantly doing favors and being asked to pitch in, in addition to handling her own sizable workload. And it was always for the same person: Rhiannon. She was well-liked and charming and had a talent for turning her crises into Dahlia's responsibility, even though they were peers. Every time Dahlia tried to set a limit, guilt—and her ingrained habit of believing she *should* be helpful and competent—overruled her inner voice. But this time, as Rhiannon asked yet again to bail her out and clean up some slides, the feeling that she was being taken advantage of overruled the anxious knot in her stomach. "I'm sorry, I can't this time. I'm stretched thin, too, and I need to focus on my own work, so I have to say no." Taken aback, Rhiannon pressed on, her voice edging with something sharp. Dahlia had *always* helped before, and she was *so* good at this stuff. "I didn't realize it was *too much* for you," she wheedled. "Rhi, I'm saying no as kindly as possible. If you continue to push it, I'll have to let our team lead know—it's just not okay to expect this of me." To her surprise, it worked! Rhiannon backed off, and Dahlia felt secure that she could protect her workload in the future if she needed to. Even though it was scary, for the first time in a long time she felt capable and confident and on a more practical level was able to actually eat her entire lunch (even if it was at her desk).

Communicating our boundary asks us to use assertive, clear, respectful communication, avoiding any blame or shame toward others. And remember: In this family, we state boundaries as "If you do X, I'll do Y," and express them as calmly and neutrally as we can, without emotions. Your boundaries are not about other people—we are not here to cajole them into living the way that you wish they would. That's paternalistic, unkind, disrespectful, and simply not what we're about here. Techniques like using "I" statements ("I feel overwhelmed when I don't have enough time to myself") empower you to express your boundaries without implicating others. The goal of stating your boundaries is to give other people an opportunity to respect your limits and give yourself explicit permission to take care of yourself if they do not.

It's often easier and most effective to state a boundary after we've already tried setting an internal boundary and communicating directly about our needs. An external boundary follows naturally as a way to reinforce what is and is not okay with you.

Let's do a little thought experiment together to see how this process builds on itself. Imagine, *por ejemplo*, that I'm at my in-laws' house for dinner. My father-in-law, Tom, is a phenomenal baker, and one of those people who shows love and care through food. There is so much goodness that comes out of his kitchen, but there's a hitch: I'm allergic to gluten, a gal with true Celiac disease. For all the years I've been part of this family, that nugget never seemed to stick, and every dinner becomes the same dance between me and Tom: He pressures me to eat and I feel bad for hurting his feelings, so I give in and nibble a breadstick, and invariably I'm sick for weeks all because I wanted to get him off my back.

Lately, though, I've been doing all this work to reclaim my sense of self and am starting to believe that my physical health is worth taking care of, even if Tom's confused or let down. Heading into dinner this Saturday, I know my limit: I do not want to eat gluten; it hurts me and makes me sick. I've also set the internal boundary that, when someone passes me the bread basket, I'm just going to hand it to the next person without taking anything. So far so good, until Tom notices that there's no bread on my plate. *Time for direct communication!* "No, thanks, Tom, I'm not going to have any tonight," I say cheerfully. It works for a minute, but before long he's begging me to try the new recipe. "It sounds delicious! But gluten makes me sick so, no, thank you!" I try again, to little success.

At this point, I've already honored my limit with that internal boundary and communicated my needs directly. I'm still being pushed to cross my limit, so it's time to set that external boundary, which sounds like "Hey, Tom! I don't eat gluten, and we've talked about how it makes me sick. I love you and I won't be pressured into something that doesn't feel right for me. If this keeps coming up, I'm going to go take some space."

How you deliver your boundary is 80 percent of the challenge. If I lose it and yell my boundary at Tom, that's not going to sound like a loving limit. Same if I seethe or roll my eyes. Folks may not be used to hearing you express a boundary, and it's true that some people will react negatively. But the goal of stating your boundary is to remind folks where you begin and they end—to remind yourself and others that *you* will be making decisions for you, not them, regardless of what has happened in the past. Try your best to speak in a calm but firm tone. Go for nonchalance if you can. Take time to regulate your nervous system if you need it, rehearse what you want to say ahead of time, and deliver it with as much neutrality and as little judgment as you can. Your goal is to take care of you with clear kindness, not to make them feel anything.

But What Do I Say?

I know from my clients that formulating boundaries can be hard to do. Even when we have a sense of our limits and what we'd like to be different, it can be hard to find words that feel natural. Boundaries are a language that we didn't learn to speak as we were growing up, and we haven't gotten much practice in adulthood either, so let's look at some more examples together:

- Hey! Please stop taking my stuff without asking, yeah? If you keep doing it, I'm going to lock my door.
- If you show up at my house without advance notice, I'm going to ask for my key back.
- I need you to stop commenting on my body. If you don't, I'm going to leave.
- I can only commit to working on this project two hours today. Let's plan accordingly, and know that even if the task runs long, I still have to leave at 4 p.m.
- If you keep cutting me off midsentence, I'm going to have to ask for some uninterrupted airtime to get my thoughts out.
- When I'm sharing painful stories from my past, I need your attention and presence. If you're unable to stay focused, I'll check in a maximum of two times and will stop sharing if you're not able to show up for this challenging conversation right now. It's painful for me and not helpful for our relationship to keep trying.
- I hear how urgent this is for you and I'm happy to help, but I'm busy until 5 p.m. today. If it can't wait until then, I won't be able to help this time.
- I need to trust that you can pick up the kids on time from school. If you can't do that, I'm going to ask that Javi's mom bring them home from now on and we'll need to have some real talk about shared responsibility.

- I understand that I messed up and you're angry with me, but I won't tolerate being yelled at or insulted. I'm going to go in the other room for a while and we'll pick this up later unless you can speak to me more respectfully.

PLAN FOR PUSHBACK

When we stop people-pleasing, well...people aren't pleased. It's the reason that so many of us don't set boundaries in the first place, and it makes a lot of sense: Not everyone is going to be thrilled that you're no longer available to walk their dog at a moment's notice, or take on that extra project, or assume blame for things that you are not at fault for.

Given the exaggerated sense of responsibility we often feel for others' emotions and well-being, folks with Emotional Outsourcing mistakenly believe that it's our job to keep them from having "negative" feelings. So we swoop in at the first hint of discomfort and shape-shift and smooth ourselves until the other person feels better. I often see this cycle kick into high gear for my clients right after they've expressed a boundary. Realizing that the other person is not, in fact, delighted at this change, my clients backtrack, soft-pedal, overexplain, and generally water down the boundary until the other person can live with it...which kinda defeats the whole purpose of setting it in the first place.

Instead, we're going to plan for pushback and decide how we would like to respond when someone tests our new boundary. Practical exercises like role-playing or journaling offer a safe space to explore and practice boundary setting and are especially helpful when you need to build muscle memory for how you'd like to respond when someone disrespects your boundary.

Let's look at an example. My client Lily was sick of her sister Mary no-showing on their plans. They'd talked about it loads of times, and when Mary bailed on dinner reservations for the third time in a row, Lily gave her a call: "Hi, so I understand something came up again, but we've talked about this. If you cancel last minute again, I'm not going to reschedule. I value our time together, but I value my time, too, and I need to know I can count on you to show up when we make plans."

"I know, I'm so, so sorry, it's just that I got caught up at work so I was home late, and then Jason started yelling at me and it was just a whole thing. You understand! But I love you, and, yes, okay, I'll do better. Promise."

"I hope you do, sis. I love you, and I love spending time with you, but I also need to take care of myself. So, seriously, if things keep going like this, I'm not going to keep making plans with you."

The next week, Mary didn't show for their sushi date and didn't even reply to Lily's "Where are you?" text until well after Lily had left the restaurant. So when Mary texted, "I'm so sorry. You just know how things are for me and I couldn't get away. Can I make it up to you next week?" Lily decided it was time to enforce her boundary. Instead of making plans that she knew full well would get canceled, Lily texted her sister back: "Sorry, M, but like I said, I can't keep making plans if you're going to cancel and no-show like this. Let's take a few weeks off."

True to form, Mary launched into a story intended to make Lily forget how hurt and upset she was at being overlooked and see things from Mary's perspective. It was stressful, but Lily was prepared for it. She put down her phone for a bit to ground herself and did a little thought work when she noticed the urge to cave and give Mary one more shot. She stayed committed to her boundary, and for the first time in a while she felt like her time was respected—by herself most of all. Who knew how things would go when she tried again in a few weeks? Worst case, she could always adjust or reaffirm her boundaries as needed.

Hard as it can be in the moment, the people in your life need to learn that you say what you mean and you mean what you say. When a boundary is new, you may have to state or enforce it a few times before it sticks. Reminding people of your boundaries is not a failure and not automatic proof that they don't care about you or that your boundary isn't okay—other people are humans too, out here managing their own insecurities and anxieties, and not memorizing your limits and boundaries doesn't mean they don't love you—it's okay to give folks the grace. And, again, my tenderoni, boundaries are not punishments: They are statements of what loving action you will take in response to someone else's actions. It is not inherently harmful to cut a conversation short, to protect your time or energy, or to follow through on what you said you would do to take care of yourself.

Most importantly, *you* need to know that you will stand up for you, that you take your needs seriously, and that you're prepared to act in loving ways to care for yourself—even and especially when others don't. Respect yourself and your relationships enough to communicate with clarity and consistency, and show everyone involved that you're not going to compromise your needs and core values just because they're uncomfortable or inconvenient for others.

All of that said, bear in mind that it is entirely up to you whether you want to enforce the consequences of a boundary or not. Healthy boundaries are adaptable, flexible, and responsive to new information. For example, if it turned out that a car accident was the reason Mary hadn't made it to their sushi date, it's up to Lily whether that changes her feelings. She might decide that this time it really wasn't Mary's fault and give it another shot or, equally, she can honor that she's still reached her limit with this pattern and needs a break, even though this latest lateness wasn't Mary's doing exactly. The choice is yours, and the only "right" decision is the one that helps you to honor yourself, your relationship, and your limits, with love toward greater interdependence and mutual compassion.

Safety First. Always.

I want to be clear that how people respond to our boundaries is highly variable, and the negative impact is more real for some than for others. That is, for folks living in marginalized identities, retaliation at work or in interpersonal relationships is a real risk and can manifest as various forms of discrimination, verbal abuse, professional repercussions, or even physical harm. That's some realness for sure—it's a complex issue tied to broader societal structures of oppression that need to be addressed for genuine equity and inclusion.

In the meantime, my love, any situation where your physical safety is at issue is *not* an appropriate moment to enforce a boundary. If the cops pull you over and yell at you to get out of the car, that is not the moment to say, "Loud voices are really stressful for me; if you continue to yell, I'm going to put in my noise-canceling headphones"... because obviously not. Same goes for situations of abuse: If trying to leave the room or the house when your husband is angry would be more likely to escalate rather than de-escalate that situation, especially if it would lead to violence, *do not* enforce that boundary. Your safety comes first. Period. Get to safety.

Asserting boundaries in a relationship goes well beyond just knowing what you need. It's a courageous act of self-love to voice those needs and ask that they be met, even when it risks causing discomfort, upset, or change. This shift from neglecting ourselves for the sake of others to prioritizing our own capacity and well-being is crucial to break the cycle of Emotional Outsourcing and move toward healthier, more balanced, and mutual relationships.

Every time you set and uphold a boundary, you teach your nervous system that it is safe to do so and that it can trust you to make good decisions for yourself. Start with the things that maybe don't sound like a lot—telling your best friend you have to leave by 9 p.m., sharing with a therapist that you're not ready to talk about that big scary thing just yet, or just trying on "no, thank you!" when you aren't interested—and work your way up to the harder conversations little by little. In this family we cheer ourselves on every step of the way, celebrating each new kitten step toward interdependence. 'Cause that's what it's all about, my loves: honoring and celebrating your true self, anchoring deep in the knowledge that because you are safe, loved, and at home with yourself, you can be in relationships without compromising on what keeps you radiant.

JOURNAL PROMPTS
EXPLORING YOUR RELATIONSHIP TO LIMITS AND BOUNDARIES

The process of setting boundaries all starts by getting familiar with our limits. We do this by noticing what makes us comfortable and uncomfortable, what feels right and what makes us feel guilty, overwhelmed, and sick to our stomachs. As you start noticing, honoring, and communicating boundaries, use these reflection questions to help you notice where you feel stuck or hesitant, as well as to imagine how clear, compassionate boundaries might help you prioritize your well-being and cultivate self-respect while maintaining connections with others.

1. Think of a recent time when you felt uncomfortable in a situation with someone else. What signs did your body give you that something didn't feel right? (For example, did your chest feel tight, did you feel anxious, or did you get a headache?)

2. Reflect on a moment when you said yes to something but later wished you had said no. What made it hard to say no in that moment, and how did you feel afterward?

3. What are some situations where you tend to overextend yourself? (For example, taking on too much at work or saying yes to plans when you're tired.) How do you feel when this happens?

...

...

...

4. Have you ever tried to communicate a boundary (even if you didn't think of it in those terms) to someone before? How did it go, and how did you feel during and after? Similarly, how were boundaries present (or not) in your family of origin?

...

...

...

5. Imagine someone crossing a small boundary, like interrupting you when you're talking. What worries come up when you imagine communicating a boundary, and how could you gently challenge those worries?

...

...

...

6. Take a moment to reflect on how you take care of and/or neglect your own needs. Are there small internal boundaries you can set to protect your energy (like turning off your phone at a certain time or not checking emails on weekends)?

...

...

7. Consider an area of your life where you wish you had more space or time for yourself. What kinds of limits could you set to create that space?

8. Think of a time when you pushed yourself to keep going even though you felt tired or stressed. What internal signs did you ignore? How might you pause and honor those signals in the future?

9. Reflect on how you feel after spending time with certain people or in specific environments. What bodily sensations arise that might indicate you've reached an internal limit, and how could you respond to those signals next time?

10. What might it feel like to honor your internal limit, even if it means stepping away or saying no to something? How could you practice self-compassion as you learn to respect your limits?

11. Reflect on a recent interaction where you felt your boundaries were crossed. What specific behaviors or actions led you to perceive a breach of your boundaries? What might you need to ask for or do to take care of yourself in the future?

....

....

....

12. Imagine an ideal scenario where your boundaries are consistently respected in this relationship. What changes would need to occur for this vision to become a reality, and what steps can you take to move closer to this outcome?

....

....

....

Conclusion

Your Favorite Life

I am so proud of you, my love. Whether you've been pausing along the way to practice and reflect, or you read all the way through to get a full lay of the land before diving in, you made it through the book and are working to teach yourself something radical and different from anything you've known. The world you grew up in showed you that you were not worthy of love and care just for being you. Your experiences with your caregivers and as a resident of a world governed by oppressive patriarchal, white-settler colonialist, and capitalist norms taught you that you were not enough. You learned that you were not safe unless you were doing, proving yourself, and tap-dancing for your lovability, and so your mind and nervous system thought that existing for others at your own expense was the only way to be. You came to believe that your value is tied to what you can produce and who you are in the eyes of others, caught in a cycle of doing the most, feeling the worst or totally numb, and pleasing everyone except yourself. Most of all, the world taught you to abandon your true self in order to source safety, worth, and belonging. It taught you that your authenticity wasn't welcome or acceptable—that your authentic thoughts, feelings, needs, wants, and experiences didn't matter.

And yet here you are, brave one, because you know deep in your heart that those stories are not true, and you're ready to give yourself permission to live a life that is big and beautiful. A life that affirms your dignity and fights for the dignity of all those around you. A life full of the radical notion that only when you care for your authenticity can you give well and care for others. Not your "best" life, not your most independent life, but your favorite life.

Your favorite life is one where you know what's real for you and what you want on your own terms. It's the life you live when you trust yourself and take care of yourself, confident that you are good and whole exactly as you are. You know what you want and need. You know what works for you in relationships and what doesn't, and you can advocate for yourself with compassion and kindness. Because you are grounded, you are able to be generous, to offer care and love to others from a full cup, without worrying about what it says about you. We get to move from a life ruled by obligation to a life with space for openhearted generosity. In our favorite lives, intention, authenticity, and regulated nervous systems run the show. They allow you to have relationships that are more generous and reciprocal than you may have ever previously known was possible.

I know this is what waits for you, my love, because I've made that journey myself.

There is a part of me that still feels bad for "complaining" about my childhood. After all, my parents took really good physical care of us: They kept really yummy Argentine food on the table, they kept us clothed for each season, our mom schlepped us to swim practice at the YMCA and gymnastics clear across town. We had every material thing we wanted... and even so, I grew up really, really, really lonely, as so many of us do with overworked, exhausted (in my case immigrant) parents trying to make their way in a (foreign) country with two little kiddos.

My parents were a product of their time and place—in our case a time and place where a brutal dictatorship held our homeland in its violent grip, where speaking out or being noticed could literally get you killed. Through no fault of their own, my emotionally immature parents grew up in systems and with personal and ancestral trauma that taught them not to have, express, or acknowledge feelings, a survival skill they passed down to me. I grew up in functional freeze believing that I—with all my gregarious, joyful, weirdo Leo energy—was way too much because the reality was that I *was* too much for my parents, given their nervous system capacity.

My father worked ridiculous hours and came home exhausted, grumpy, and hangry, and my mother very clearly resented her whole wife-and-mother gig, constantly telling us just how much she suffered for us. My parents didn't know how to handle it when my overwhelming delight had me skipping around the house, giggles at the fullest volume, while they had left their joy back home on the beach in Argentina.

I felt like a burden and a bother, unacceptable, a problem, like I was always wrong and messing up, and like my emotions were dangerous (after all, they could make people sad or mad, which was scary for sure). I was untethered—a depressed and lonely twelve-year-old with tummy troubles, constantly searching for solid ground in other people, places, and things in a family and a country where I felt like I didn't belong. Believing deep inside me that I wasn't worthy of love and care, that my opinions didn't matter, my understanding of the world just plain wrong (having heard that at home 473 times), I learned to shove my authentic self down, down, down and took on the persona of the people I was around—later mostly the person I was dating, whose interests became mine in the blink of an eye.

I would contort myself to please my date, to make her happy, to win her praise. I had no idea I was living codependently, that I was people-pleasing and seeking safety in others' approval of me. I was desperate for a place to moor the boat of my rich inner life, and I'd become whoever I needed to be to feel accepted. Reenacting, like we do, I dated meanie after meanie who had no real interest in seeing me and def no interest in respecting me, and when I finally dated someone truly, deeply kind, I found the whole thing so boring I was itching to get out by the second date—but moved in with her anyway.

By the time I entered my twenties, I was deep in functional freeze—excelling at school, getting fancy degrees, studying medicine to attempt to gain approval in the eyes of my unapproving father (whom I loved more than myself), cutting ties and moving towns without batting an eye (which is easy to do when you feel like you don't matter to anyone), completely numb to my own desires, wants, needs, preferences. Though I was keenly aware of my own chronic irritation, annoyance, frustration with, and resentment in these endless lousy relationships, there was a part of me (whom I didn't discover until many years later) who believed that I was not worthy of having what I actually wanted, a part that implored me to settle. If you said you liked me, I was yours, regardless of how I felt... if I even really knew how I felt at all.

The apex (or nadir, however you wanna look at it) of all of this was a lousy relationship turned abusive first marriage. It was a hot mess of dysfunction from the jump: I was repulsed by their lack of self-care and general uncleanliness, their unkempt space and clothes. I was deeply turned off by their profound entitlement, who they were and how they lived... but they asked me out, so who was I to say no? A few months in I got the support I needed to tell them I wasn't interested, that it was over and I was moving on—and I got horrifyingly sick the next day. I was admitted to the hospital for four days (a very long time indeed for a healthy athletic woman in her early thirties) and they were the only person who stayed by my side, getting me food and drinks, sleeping on a recliner in my hospital room—they were also the only person I told, not even considering calling my friends because thoughts like "Call Luca and Felice, Suneye and Kelly" didn't even cross my mind, I was so used to going it alone and not being a bother. My dad rushed to my side and sat in my hospital room for the day, and true to form he didn't talk to me the whole time, mostly staring into the middle distance, asking nothing about my life, not interacting with me in any substantive way. He was functioning at the top of his capacity, which I don't fault him for, but it left me feeling more lost and alone than had he not come to see me. My mother's comfort, meanwhile, was never a consideration—not because she didn't care, but because I knew that being vulnerable around her never felt safe. Emotionally, she was still figuring out how to tend to her own needs in a mature way, and I had learned long ago that in moments like this, I'd end up managing her feelings or temper tantrums instead of receiving care myself. Meanwhile, this person, this date I didn't want to date anymore, was *physically there*—which was more than I thought I could expect from anyone at that point—and even though most of me wanted to get as far from them as possible, a very little girl inside me, a young and scared inner child, said, *Well, they're here, aren't they? Might as well settle and take what we can get—it's not like anyone better is out there*... And so I stayed. Relationship Magical Realism to the max.

Years later we married—not because I actually wanted to, but because they asked, and the morning of my wedding I told my then best friend I wanted out. I'll never forget her looking me right in the eyes and saying, "That train has left the station." My spouse had a terrible temper, serious anger issues, and the smallest inconvenience or request for them to change behavior led to hours of them screaming, towering over me while I cowered in the bed, begging and pleading them to stop. They had no off button and wouldn't back down until I took full responsibility for whatever had happened or had bothered them by apologizing for things I hadn't done or going back on any ask, saying things like "You're right, I shouldn't have asked you to help with the dishes—I'm so so so sorry." They told me my hormones were unbalanced and I was probably bipolar or a thousand other diagnoses they would pull out of thin air to manipulate me, that it was my "craziness" and "moodiness" that were the problem . . . accusations I had ruled out by licensed medical doctors and psychologists who found me physically and mentally competent—not diagnosable, just stuck. I was living between a rock and a hard place—staying for the hints of potential happiness while being utterly beaten down by the day-to-day, my poor nervous system fully unmoored.

There was constant gaslighting, blaming, shaming, attempts to convince me that they did so much around the house, and I was a "bitch" and a "nag" for saying otherwise—it was always all my fault, always. If I did something so thoughtless and terrible as to ask them to participate in the housework, I'd be hearing about it—often until three or four in the morning, though I had to be up at six thirty to start my day as primary care provider to hundreds of New Yorkers. A multimillionaire from what they called "truly opulent wealth," they insisted I pay for everything and refused to pay me back. It became evident that the stupidest thing I could do was to share what I was thinking with them, to ask them to do anything to help me or the household, to have an opinion or thought other than to agree with them. I went so far as to get a little tattoo on the inside of my left middle finger—two dots to remind me "don't speak" because it wasn't worth it. It never ended well. I was lonely, isolated, and scared to talk about just how bad it was. I kept shaming myself, embarrassed because "I should know better."

Suffering so deeply at home, desperate for change and for the constant stress and fighting to end, I went to therapist after therapist, looking for someone to "fix me." All I heard from my spouse was that I was 100 percent the problem—a story I found easy to believe given my scapegoat upbringing. I even fired the best therapist I'd ever had for having the audacity to say that maybe, just maybe, I wasn't the whole problem . . . but the thought stayed with me long after I left her office.

I had spent so many years as the identified patient, meditating, praying, moving my body, eating well, doing breathwork and somatic work, and spending hours in grimy church basements trying to figure out what was wrong with me, that it was revolutionary to realize that I was not, in fact, *the entire problem*—and that it was high time to rid myself of the causes and conditions of my suffering, and to reclaim my life for me.

With the help of some amazing friends and a lot of thought work, somatic work, and nervous system regulation coaching, I was able to find my footing once more, and to come face to face with that part that kept me stuck and settling—the part that whispered, *This is as good as it gets. Don't rock the boat.* The part that equated discomfort with danger, that had learned long ago to prioritize stability over self-expansion. And slowly, with patience and practice, I learned to listen without obeying, to soothe my system without silencing myself, and to step into the life I actually wanted, rather than the one I thought I had to accept.

I left that relationship, went home to Argentina to reconnect with my roots and *mi tierra*, and came back to New York ready to live life on my own terms. I used the same tools that I've taught you in this book—cultivating compassionate awareness of who I really was, engaging in somatic practices and thought work, and using boundaries to honor my limits—to cultivate a deep, internal sense of worth that no one else could give or take away.

It's rarely easy to look at your past and your present with clear eyes, but out of all that uncomfortable growth came the clarity that nobody could or should ever be my anchor in life—except me. Self-love, self-trust, and interdependent living in community are the answer. No more hitching myself to someone who was supposed to validate me and make me happy. No more handing over my sense of safety to anyone or anything. With time and practice, I came to believe in my self: the gal who had done all the challenging work, who had named her limits and kept pushing for her own survival. A woman who is a direct and amazing communicator, a generous partner who is not a nag, a person with a balanced mind in a sound body whose opinion really does matter and is worth listening to.

These days, I'm able to validate myself, rather than depending on others to tell me that I'm worthwhile and lovable. I can take a compliment (rather than brushing it away like I used to). I can ask for and receive help. I can show up for myself, recognizing my own limits, boundaries, wants, needs, and desires. And mostly, now I live my life toward interdependence—showing up for community, connection, and collective liberation any chance I can.

I owe it all to the challenging, terrifying, amazing work of overcoming Emotional Outsourcing that I find myself now, deeply and truly, madly in love, married to the most amazing woman (human!) I've ever met, experiencing unrivaled joy, peace, stability, and profound growth each and every day with Billey Albina, held by a beloved community of friends who are truly my family, who I'm deeply interdependent with.

~~~

My love, our most essential human task is to meet life in our full authenticity from our wide-open heart. And, really, what better purpose can we have in our lives than to know ourselves well and to share the glorious person that we are with other people? This is what we're healing for, *mi amor.* For more joy, more magic, more presence, more connection, more *love.* Emotional Outsourcing ends when we know that we are safe and loved and at home with
~~~

ourselves, no matter what, and are able to meet the world from that energy, unbothered by others' shenanigans.

True connection isn't about control or fixing; it's about mutual support, trust, and respect, grounded in our wholeness—something my wife, Billey (the truest love of my life), once called "mutuosity"—a portmanteau of "mutuality" and "reciprocity"—which has stuck as the bedrock of our marriage and the connective joy of every relationship in my life. Of course, our transformation from living for others at our own expense to living in mutuosity with our loved ones doesn't happen overnight. We pay a lot of lip service to the idea that healing takes time, but rarely do we talk about what's in that process. I wish that I could wave a magic wand that would rewire your Emotional Outsourcing in a snap, my darling, but the good stuff rarely happens like that.

Instead, it starts with the little things: moments of mindfulness and noticing that your body is talking to you and getting curious about what it has to say. A flicker in your mind that you didn't actually want to say yes to some new obligation or event after all, and a choice to do it differently next time. As you continue to counteract your Emotional Outsourcing habits with new self- and community-loving habits, I want you to know that the healing process is less a journey from Point A to Point B and more like a pendulum swinging from one end to another, back and forth, slowly coming to settle at peace in the middle. As you invite somatics, thought work, and loving limits into your daily life, you might swing from where you started in Emotional Outsourcing, all the way to the other side, where we are rigidly protective of our new self. Any ask is too much. We guard our window of capacity with vigilance, as if it was the crown jewels. Where before the line between you and the world didn't exist, now you might temporarily live in a fortress guarding your nervous system, your energy, and your nascent self with everything you've got.

In other words, we're very likely to overcorrect at first, because *of course* we will. I see my clients judge themselves, lose steam, and beat themselves up for not getting it exactly right the first time or for being too rigid. And I remind them that healing is iterative. "Getting it right" is just an old perfectionist story, and we don't have to believe it. Instead, I want to normalize for you this process of pendulation. Over the course of your journey, you will swing back and forth between those codependent and independent poles, mellowing a bit each time. Slowly, slowly, swing by swing, we pendulate closer to that grounded interdependence that we deserve. Don't measure your progress by whether you're in "perfect harmony" with everyone, but rather by how easily and how often you're able to step into ways of being that feel better and serve you more. This is what we mean when we say that healing is nonlinear, my love. Life happens, healing happens, and absolutely none of it happens in a "perfect" progression.

What is so exciting, my love, is that you now have the tools to create your favorite life. You get to move through your days knowing that you matter. You get to know what you need and can make choices to meet that need. You get to know how you feel in your body and take loving action to shift that nervous system experience when you need and want to. The ways you've healed will open you to relationships and opportunities you may never have ever imagined. You may even be lucky enough to see the impact of your healing on a friend, child, or loved one—it's hard to describe the joy of watching how your own work to show up for yourself and others can inspire someone else to trust their authenticity, too. Because while the struggle is ancestral, carried in bone and breath, so are wisdom, resilience, and the joy that is yours to claim.

Throughout your journey, I humbly insist that you give yourself patience and step into radical acceptance of the fact that we are never, ever "done" growing as people, and I think that's beautiful! Our brains, minds, and hearts can always evolve, can always shift, can always learn new things and adapt. New situations, opportunities, life stages, people, desires, challenges, needs—you'll get to navigate them all. And this time, you won't be stuck because you know how to

- see yourself in context, with compassion for how little you was impacted by your caregivers and oppressive social systems;
- attune to your nervous system and use somatic practices to source safety and expand your window of capacity;
- choose thoughts that bring the results you want and rewire the habitual reactions that no longer serve you; and
- honor your dignity and protect your limits by setting boundaries and lovingly communicating your needs.

In other words, you won't have to default to the codependent, perfectionist, people-pleasing habits that have been running your life. You have the tools you need to choose, for yourself, how you'd like to handle whatever life brings: a new job, town, baby, divorce, haircut, partner, identity, illness, loss, achievement—you get to braid it all into your favorite life.

Whenever you feel lost, overwhelmed, angry, frustrated, or stuck, pause and come back to your body. Orient, ground, breathe—do what we do here in this *familia* to tend to our nervous systems. Counteract the story that you have to heal exactly "right" the first time by getting curious about the perfectionism, scarcity, and self-judgment that are coming up for you in that moment.

Most of all, my love, I want you to remember that there is nothing wrong with you. Nothing at all. *Nada*. Not one single thing. You adopted the skills you needed to survive, and that served you well for a time. You are not broken and you never were. You are here with me today just as whole and beautiful and worthy of love as you have always been, Emotional Outsourcing habits and all. And I am so excited to see the ways you choose to heal and to build a life that proves that to you every single day. Until then, visit with this book as often as you need to. Come join us on Instagram at @beatrizvictoriaalbinanp or at www.beatrizalbina.com, seek support and community wherever feels good for you, and never forget: You are enough—you always have been.

You are safe.
You are held.
You are loved.
And when one of us heals
we help heal the World.

Appendix A

Nervous System Arousal Levels and Tracker

NERVOUS SYSTEM AROUSAL LEVELS

Dorsal (shut down)

-10 = Complete shutdown. Inability to engage with surroundings, despair, numbness and heaviness in the limbs, cold or clammy skin

-8 to -9 = Moderate shutdown. Low energy, feeling disconnected from others, lack of motivation, dulled physical sensations

-5 to -7 = Mild shutdown. Difficulty concentrating, avoiding social interaction, decreased interest in activities, mild aches or pains, general fatigue

-2 to -4 = Slightly below calm. Low enthusiasm

-1 = Near calm but slightly withdrawn. Mild disconnection or a sense of being "off" or disengaged; energy is still balanced, but there's a slight withdrawal from full engagement; you might feel a tinge of isolation or fatigue creeping in, perhaps a desire to be alone but not from a place of overwhelm; there's still functionality, but with a subtle pull toward retreat or rest

Ventral Vagal (safe and social)

0 = Calm and relaxed. Balanced and present, consistent energy, steady breathing, normal heart rate, sensation of lightness or buoyancy

Sympathetic (fight or flight)

1 = Near calm but slightly activated. Slight increase in energy, vigilance, and muscle tension; mild undercurrent of restlessness; fidgeting or feeling a touch more reactive to environment

2 to 4 = Mild activation. Increased alertness, elevated heart rate, "on edge" but manageable, neck and shoulder tension

5 to 7 = Moderate activation. Noticeable anxiety, difficulty concentrating, feeling overwhelmed, sweating, tension in chest

8 to 9 = High activation. High levels of panic and anxiety, irritability or anger, racing thoughts, shaking, shortness of breath, pounding heart

10 = Extreme activation. Intense panic or terror, chest pain, hyperventilation, dizziness, urge to escape or aggressive behavior, extreme sensitivity to noise or touch

Nervous System Arousal/State Tracker

What Did I Feel in My Nervous System When...

Situation

....

Nervous System State

-10 -9 -8 -7 -6 -5 -4 -3 -2 -1 0 1 2 3 4 5 6 7 8 9 10

Situation

....

Nervous System State

-10 -9 -8 -7 -6 -5 -4 -3 -2 -1 0 1 2 3 4 5 6 7 8 9 10

Situation

....

Nervous System State

-10 -9 -8 -7 -6 -5 -4 -3 -2 -1 0 1 2 3 4 5 6 7 8 9 10

Situation

....

Nervous System State

-10 -9 -8 -7 -6 -5 -4 -3 -2 -1 0 1 2 3 4 5 6 7 8 9 10

Situation

....

Nervous System State

-10 -9 -8 -7 -6 -5 -4 -3 -2 -1 0 1 2 3 4 5 6 7 8 9 10

If you'd prefer a printable version of this tracker, you can find one on my website at www.beatrizalbina.com/statetracker.

Appendix B

Thought Work Protocol Worksheet

While I often recommend using a journal to do thought work, I know that many of my clients have valued having a clear structure and quick reminders to guide them through all five steps, so I created this Thought Work Protocol Worksheet to support you. If you'd like a printable version of this worksheet, you can download one from my website, www.beatrizalbina.com/thoughtworkprotocol.

Thought Work Protocol

Date: ....

Observation *(bare-bones, court-admissible facts, no adjectives or adverbs)*

....

....

....

....

....

....

....

Interpretation *(reactions, automatic thoughts; what meaning am I making? nervous system state):*

....

....

....

....

Feeling *(emotions and bodily sensations)*

....

....

....

....

....

....

Actions *(what I did/didn't do)*

....

....

....

....

....

....

Result *(what was the outcome of those actions in* ***my*** *life?)*

....

....

....

....

....

....

....

....

....

After completing the Thought Work Protocol Worksheet to understand your think-feel-act cycle in that moment, reflect on the following questions:

- *Does this result serve me? In what ways?*
- *Would a different result serve me better? How so? What result am I hoping for?*
- *What bridge thought could take me closer to the result I hope for?*

Acknowledgments

Writing a book may be a solitary act, but it is never done alone. This work is a reflection of every conversation, every shared breath, every moment of connection that shaped my thinking and deepened my understanding of what it means to be human.

To my wife, Billey Albina—your love is both liberatory and generative, a steady presence that makes everything possible. You reminded me, again and again, that my words matter, that my voice is worth hearing, that rest is as essential to creation as the work itself. Thank you for the cups of tea and yerba mate, the patience, the laughter, and the unwavering belief that I could write this book. I love you beyond words. Thank you for showing me what embodied interdependence truly looks and feels like.

To my dear friend Kara Loewentheil, without whom my coaching career and this book would not exist in their current form. Thank you for yelling at me for over a decade, and for inviting me to yours for the holidays when I found myself so alone. I'm so grateful for your love and friendship, and for the ways you modeled what's possible, and pushed me to step it up.

To Dr. Suneye Koohsari, MD, DBOM, for loving me and being a rock of sanity, sass, and sarcasm in my life—forever your DM, there is no one I'd rather eat dumplings with than you, DA-R. *Para* Juana Berinstein, *por tu aguda inteligencia, tu claridad implacable y tu mirada precisa que siempre va al núcleo de las cosas. Por más de veinte años de conversaciones de corazón, gracias por tu apoyo inquebrantable y por caminar a mi lado en este camino.*

To my *hermanas* Sara Fisk and Judith Gaton, for always having my back and loving me up when I felt most *locquita*. For coaching me with wisdom and heart, checking my models with precision, reading drafts with care, and reminding me—always—to laugh through it all.

To Jules Netherland—this book would not exist without you. From the very beginning, sitting cross-legged on your apartment floor mapping out the bones of this work, you have been a steady source of support, love, care, brilliance, and friendship. Thank you for believing in me, for holding space, and for helping me bring this book to life. And thank you for being as formatting obsessed as I am. Every, single, comma, in, this, book, I, dedicate, to, you.

To my chosen family and dearest friends—thank you for witnessing me, holding me, and reflecting my own wisdom back to me when I needed it most. To those who listened to my spirals, read early drafts, and reminded me to touch grass when I got too deep in my head, I am forever grateful. Your love and presence are the soil in which this book was able to take root. Andrea Mignolo—*boluda, te adoro*—thank you for being my *hermana* since way back in the nineties, thanks for being my somatics-sister, and yes—Baldwin forever! Here's to Montevideo. Karen Alroy and Christina Starr—you two have been a steady rock of love and support going back over twenty years and I'm so grateful for your companionship all this time and especially in the darkness of the Upstate Years. To Rob Israel for always having a bucket ready when I need it—love you, brother, mean it. To Timmy Paul Ryan—my Banana Boat forever—love you big time, mean it. To everyone in the Ferns who put up with me in my twenties and thirties and modeled what was possible. To Jessie Gallogaly, my first friend in the U.S.—love you, bunnygirl. To everyone at the

San Francisco Zen Center Hospice who taught me so much about living by teaching me about dying. And of course, thank you to Frances (Frankie Bacon) The Bestest Dog Ever, Idgie and Moxie Cats and my newest love, Wade Stitious Cat (because in this household we're not SuperStitious, but when we bring an all-black cat into this witchy house, turns out we are a *little bit Stitious*). And to every friend I don't have space to name, know that I love you big time and am grateful for everything.

To my teachers, mentors, and guides—those who taught me, challenged me, and expanded my thinking in ways that made this work possible. Your wisdom lives in these pages, woven into every insight, every invitation to a deeper way of being. Thank you for showing me that knowledge is meant to be lived, not just learned. Specifically I want to thank Sam Grabel, my slam poetry mentor in the nineties, Dr. Robert, my high school English teacher at Classical High School; Dr. Steven Volk and Dr. Ana Cara, my advisors at Oberlin; Dr. Richard Clapp, Laura Orlando, and Abby Rockefeller—my teachers, mentors, and pals at Boston University. You nerds modeled the potent, world-changing power of geeking out on the things that turn your brain on, and I can't tell you how endlessly and forever grateful I am to be the nerd I am, thanks to you all (and *Because Science*).

To my incredible team—to Hannah Robinson, who encouraged me to write this book and midwifed it into existence. I couldn't have done it without you HannitaLinda! Richelle Fredson, you not only led me through the proposal process, you've held my hand ever since and I'm so grateful—you're really good at your job. Thanks of course to Diana Ventimiglia, who inherited this book and cheered it on, and to my agent, Wendy Sherman, for all that you did along the way. To Cher Hale, my publicist of many years, for your brilliance, dedication, and unwavering belief in my work. Thank you for championing my voice and making sure it reaches the people who need it most. Larissa Zozula and the whole *Feminist*

Wellness team—I'm so grateful for your support—couldn't keep the ship afloat without you.

To everyone at Balance who helped shape this book into its fullest form, and everyone who worked tirelessly to bring it into the world. Your skill, care, and dedication are deeply felt, and I am beyond grateful.

To my family of origin—thank you for crossing continents and reshaping your lives, for leaving behind the familiar to build a new life, for your own dreams and for the family's future. I know you did the best you could with what you had, and for that, I hold gratitude. *Y para Tía Bichi, por mostrarme lo que realmente es el amor incondicional.*

To the Feminist Wellness, Anchored, and Somatic Studio communities—those who have listened to the podcast, taken my courses, read my words, and engaged in this work with open hearts and minds. You are the reason this book exists. Your questions, your insights, your courage in showing up for yourselves and your healing have shaped this work in ways I could never fully express. Thank you for trusting me to walk alongside you.

Mil gracias a Fito Páez, Celeste Carballo, Charly García y tantos músicos del Rock Nacional Argentino—me acompañaron sin saberlo en tantas largas noches de escribir y escribir. Ser una piba argentina tan lejos de casa y tener sus voces en mi oído ha sido un bálsamo, un pedacito de hogar que me ha dado vida.

And finally, to the Land, to Pachamama, to my ancestors, to all the thinkers and writers and radical dreamers who came before me, to the feminist theorists who shaped me in my teens, twenties, and since—Audre Lorde, Adrienne Rich, bell hooks, Gloria Anzaldúa, María Lugones, June Jordan, and so many more—your words cracked me open and rewrote my world. Thank you for the wisdom, the resilience, the whispers of encouragement that carried me through. I am the feminist and writer I am today thanks to you.

This book is not mine alone. It belongs to every person who has ever longed to step out of the tangle of Emotional Outsourcing and into the fullness of their own life. May it be a lantern in the dark, a gentle hand on your back, a reminder that you are already whole, and you deserve nothing less than amazing things in this life—go get 'em, you tender little ravioli you!

Notes

Chapter 1: What Is Emotional Outsourcing?

1. Greg E. Dear, Beverley M. Roberts, and T. Ian K. Hassall, "The Holyoake Codependency Index: A Measure of Codependency," *Journal of Clinical Psychology* 54, no. 1 (1998): 63–73.
2. Robert J. Rotunda, Stephen F. West, and Diana L. O'Farrell, "Enabling Behavior in a Clinical Sample of Alcohol-Dependent Clients and Their Partners," *Journal of Substance Abuse Treatment* 26, no. 4 (2004): 269–276; Greg E. Dear and Gavan P. Roberts, "The Relationships between Codependency and Femininity and Masculinity," *Sex Roles* 38, no. 9–10 (1998): 901–913.
3. Emeran A. Mayer, "The Neurobiology of Stress and Gastrointestinal Disease," *Gut* 47, no. 6 (2000): 861–869.
4. Shounak Baksi and Ajay Pradhan, "Thyroid Hormone: Sex-Dependent Role in Nervous System Regulation and Disease," *Biology of Sex Differences* 12, no. 1 (2021): 25, https://doi.org/10.1186/s13293-021-00367-2; George P. Chrousos, "Stress and Disorders of the Stress System," *Nature Reviews Endocrinology* 5, no. 7 (2009): 374–381.
5. Suzanne C. Segerstrom and Gregory E. Miller, "Psychological Stress and the Human Immune System: A Meta-Analytic Study of 30 Years of Inquiry," *Psychological Bulletin* 130, no. 4 (2004): 601–630; Alan Rozanski, James A. Blumenthal, and Jonathan D. Kaplan, "Impact of Psychological Factors on the Pathogenesis of Cardiovascular Disease and Implications for Therapy," *Circulation* 99, no. 16 (1999): 2192–2217.
6. Charles M. Morin and Ruth Benca, "Chronic Insomnia," *Lancet* 379, no. 9821 (2012): 1129–1141.
7. Firdaus S. Dhabhar, "Effects of Stress on Immune Function: The Good, the Bad, and the Beautiful," *Immunologic Research* 58, no. 2–3 (2014): 193–210.
8. Robert Kirkpatrick, "Codependency: A Critical Review," *Alcoholism Treatment Quarterly* 8, no. 1 (1991): 29–36.
9. Audre Lorde, *A Burst of Light* (Mineola, NY: Dover Publications, 2017), epilogue, Libby.
10. Audre Lorde, *Sister Outsider: Essays and Speeches* (Berkeley, CA: Ten Speed Press, 2007), 146.

Chapter 2: The Origin of Your Self-Story

1. Barbara A. Morrongiello, Susan K. Zdzieborski, and Mike Normand, "Parents' Home-Safety Practices to Prevent Injuries during Infancy," *Journal of Pediatric Psychology* 47, no. 6 (2022): 687–697; Adriana Vieira Mello, Lilian Gonçalves Ferreira, and Marisa Schmitz de Moraes, "Child Safety from the Perspective of Essential Needs," *Child and Adolescent Social Work Journal* 31, no. 3 (2014): 219–232; Hyun-Jin Kim, Sung-Eun Hong,

and Mi-Jung Jang, "Analysis of Research on Interventions for the Prevention of Safety Accidents Involving Infants," *International Journal of Environmental Research and Public Health* 19, no. 9 (2022): 5506.

2. Esther M. Leerkes, A. Nayena Blankson, and Marion O'Brien, "Differential Effects of Maternal Sensitivity to Infant Distress and Nondistress on Social-Emotional Functioning," *Child Development* 80, no. 3 (2009): 762–775; Daniel N. Stern, *The Interpersonal World of the Infant: A View from Psychoanalysis and Developmental Psychology* (London: Karnac Books, 1998), 27; Allan N. Schore, "Effects of a Secure Attachment Relationship on Right Brain Development, Affect Regulation, and Infant Mental Health," *Infant Mental Health Journal* 22, no. 1–2 (2001): 4.
3. Stern, *The Interpersonal World of the Infant*; Schore, "Effects of a Secure Attachment Relationship," 38–39.
4. Stephen W. Porges, *The Polyvagal Theory: Neurophysiological Foundations of Emotions, Attachment, Communication, and Self-Regulation*, 1st ed. Norton Series on Interpersonal Neurobiology (New York: W.W. Norton, 2011).
5. C. Rees, "Childhood Attachment," *British Journal of General Practice* 57, no. 544 (2007): 920–922.
6. Susan H. Landry, Karen E. Smith, and Paul R. Swank, "Responsive Parenting: Establishing Early Foundations for Social, Communication, and Independent Problem-Solving Skills," *Developmental Psychology* 42, no. 4 (2006): 627–642.
7. John Bowlby, *Attachment and Loss*, vol. 1, *Attachment* (London: Pimlico, 1997).
8. Mary D.S. Ainsworth, Mary C. Blehar, Everett Waters, and Sally Wall, *Patterns of Attachment: A Psychological Study of the Strange Situation* (Hillsdale, NJ: Lawrence Erlbaum Associates, 1978).
9. Norman Doidge, *The Brain That Changes Itself: Stories of Personal Triumph from the Frontiers of Brain Science* (New York: Viking, 2007).
10. Judy Ho, *The New Rules of Attachment: How to Heal Your Relationships, Reparent Your Inner Child, and Secure Your Life Vision* (New York: Hachette Book Group, 2024).
11. Daniel A. Hughes, *Building the Bonds of Attachment: Awakening Love in Deeply Traumatized Children*, 2nd ed. (Lanham, MD: Rowman & Littlefield, 2006).
12. Donald W. Winnicott, "Ego Distortion in Terms of True and False Self," in *The Maturational Processes and the Facilitating Environment: Studies in the Theory of Emotional Development*, 1st ed. (London: Routledge, 2018), 140–152.
13. Vincent J. Felitti, R.F. Anda, D. Nordenberg, D.F. Williamson, A.M. Spitz, V. Edwards, et al., "Relationship of Childhood Abuse and Household Dysfunction to Many of the Leading Causes of Death in Adults: The Adverse Childhood Experiences (ACE) Study," *American Journal of Preventive Medicine* 14, no. 4 (1998): 245–258.
14. Diana Baumrind, "Child Care Practices Anteceding Three Patterns of Preschool Behavior," *Genetic Psychology Monographs* 75, no. 1 (1967): 43-88.
15. Eleanor E. Maccoby and John A. Martin, "Socialization in the Context of the Family: Parent-Child Interaction," in *Handbook of Child Psychology*, 4th ed., ed. P.H. Mussen, vol. 4, *Socialization, Personality, and Social Development*, ed. E.M. Hetherington (New York: Wiley, 1983), 1–101.
16. Diana Baumrind, "Effects of Authoritarian Parenting on Child Behavior," *Child Development* 37, no. 4 (1966): 887–907.
17. Maccoby and Martin, "Socialization in the Context of the Family."
18. Patricia McKinsey Crittenden and Andrea Landini, *Assessing Adult Attachment: A Dynamic-Maturational Approach to Discourse Analysis* (New York: W.W. Norton, 2011).

19. Neil Montgomery, *The Nurtured Heart Approach to Parenting: A Resource for Parents and Therapists* (Tucson, AZ: Children's Success Foundation, 2010).
20. Ivan Boszormenyi-Nagy and Geraldine M. Spark, *Invisible Loyalties: Reciprocity in Intergenerational Family Therapy* (Hagerstown, MD: Harper & Row, 1973).
21. Gregory J. Jurkovic, *The Plight of the Parentified Child* (New York: Brunner/Mazel, 1997); Nancy D. Chase, *Burdened Children: Theory, Research, and Treatment of Parentification* (Thousand Oaks, CA: Sage Publications, 1999).
22. Lisa Damour, *Under Pressure: Confronting the Epidemic of Stress and Anxiety in Girls* (New York: Ballantine Books, 2019); Constance P. Rossmann and Thomas D. Yoder, "Adult Success and Its Predictors as Related to Early Childhood Chores," *Journal of Child and Family Studies* (2017); Eva H. Telzer and Andrew J. Fuligni, "Daily Family Assistance and the Psychological Well-Being of Adolescents from Latin American, Asian, and European Backgrounds," *Developmental Psychology* 45, no. 4 (2009): 1177–1189.
23. Gregory Miller and Edith Chen, "The Biological Residue of Childhood Poverty," *Child Development Perspectives* 8, no. 2 (2014): 67–73.
24. Daniel J. Siegel and Tina Payne Bryson, *The Whole-Brain Child: 12 Revolutionary Strategies to Nurture Your Child's Developing Mind* (New York: Bantam Books, 2011); Michael T. Kinsella and David E. Monkhouse, "Gaslighting as a Form of Psychological Abuse," *Psychiatry Research* 303 (2021): 114–121, https://doi.org/10.1016/j.psychres2021; Brené Brown, *The Gifts of Imperfection: Let Go of Who You Think You're Supposed to Be and Embrace Who You Are* (Center City, MN: Hazelden Publishing, 2010).
25. Mary Main and Judith Solomon, "Discovery of an Insecure-Disorganized/Disoriented Attachment Pattern," in *Affective Development in Infancy*, ed. T.B. Brazelton and M.W. Yogman (Westport, CT: Ablex Publishing Corporation, 1986), 95–124.
26. Ronald P. Rohner, "Introduction to Interpersonal Acceptance–Rejection Theory (IPAR-Theory) and Evidence," *Online Readings in Psychology and Culture* 6, no. 1 (2016).
27. Allan N. Schore, "The Effects of Early Relational Trauma on Right Brain Development, Affect Regulation, and Infant Mental Health," *Infant Mental Health Journal* 22, no. 1–2 (2001): 201–269, https://doi.org/10.1002/imhj.1009.
28. Peter Fonagy and Mary Target, "Attachment and Reflective Function: Their Role in Self-Organization," *Development and Psychopathology* 9, no. 4 (1997): 679–700, https://doi.org/10.1017/S0954579497001399.
29. Mary Main and Judith Solomon, "Procedures for Identifying Infants as Disorganized/Disoriented During the Ainsworth Strange Situation," in *Attachment in the Preschool Years: Theory, Research, and Intervention*, ed. Mark T. Greenberg, Dante Cicchetti, and E. Mark Cummings (Chicago: University of Chicago Press, 1990), 121–160; David Luxton, "The Effects of Inconsistent Parenting on the Development of Uncertain Self-Esteem and Depression Vulnerability," 2007; Bessel A. van der Kolk, *The Body Keeps the Score: Brain, Mind, and Body in the Healing of Trauma* (New York: Penguin Books, 2014); John Bowlby, *Attachment and Loss: Volume I* (New York: Basic Books, 1969); Leon Festinger, *A Theory of Cognitive Dissonance* (Stanford, CA: Stanford University Press, 1957).
30. Jay Belsky, Laurence Steinberg, and Patricia Draper, "Childhood Experience, Interpersonal Development, and Reproductive Strategy: An Evolutionary Theory of Socialization," *Child Development* 62, no. 4 (1991): 647, https://doi.org/10.2307/1131166.

Chapter 3: The Trap of Functional Freeze

1. Stephen W. Porges and S.A. Furman, "The Early Development of the Autonomic Nervous System Provides a Neural Platform for Social Behavior: A Polyvagal Perspective,"

Infant and Child Development 20, no. 1 (2011): 106–118, https://doi.org/10.1002/icd.688; Tiffany Field and Miguel Diego, "Vagal Activity, Early Growth, and Emotional Development," *Infant Behavior and Development* 31, no. 3 (2008): 361–373, https://doi.org/10.1016/j.infbeh.2007.12.008.

2. N.B. Schmidt, J.A. Richey, M.J. Zvolensky, and J.K. Maner, "Exploring Human Freeze Responses to a Threat Stressor," *Journal of Behavior Therapy and Experimental Psychiatry* 39, no. 3 (2008): 292–304, https://doi.org/10.1016/j.jbtep.2007.08.002.
3. Pete Walker, *Complex PTSD: From Surviving to Thriving* (Lafayette, CA: Azure Coyote, 2013).
4. Stephen W. Porges, *The Polyvagal Theory: The Evolutionary Origins of Wellness and Trauma* (New York: W.W. Norton, 2011), 32; Deb Dana, *Polyvagal Theory in Therapy: Engaging the Rhythm of Regulation* (New York: W.W. Norton, 2018), 45; Peter A. Levine and Ann Frederick, *Healing Trauma: A Pioneering Program for Restoring the Wisdom of Your Body* (Boulder, CO: Sounds True, 1997), 66.
5. Stephen Porges, "Neuroception: A Subconscious System for Detecting Threats and Safety," *Zero to Three* 24, no. 5 (2004): 19–24.
6. Stephen W. Porges, "Polyvagal Theory: A Science of Safety," *Frontiers in Psychology* 10 (2019), https://www.frontiersin.org/articles/10.3389/fpsyg.2019.02646/full; "What Is the Polyvagal Theory?," Polyvagal Institute, accessed September 5, 2024, https://www.polyvagalinstitute.org/whatispolyvagaltheory.
7. S.W. Porges, "Orienting in a Defensive World: Mammalian Modifications of Our Evolutionary Heritage: A Polyvagal Theory," *Psychophysiology* 32, no. 4 (1995): 301–318; S.W. Porges, "The Polyvagal Theory: Phylogenetic Substrates of a Social Nervous System," *International Journal of Psychophysiology* 42, no. 2 (2001): 123–146; S.W. Porges, "The Polyvagal Perspective," *Biological Psychology* 74, no. 2 (2007): 116–143.
8. Deb Dana, *Polyvagal Theory in Therapy: Engaging the Rhythm of Regulation* (New York: W.W. Norton, 2018); F.R. Amthor, Chapter 18: Autonomic Nervous System: Sympathetic, Parasympathetic, & Enteric, in F.R. Amthor, A.B. Theibert, D.G. Standaert, and E.D. Roberson, eds., *Essentials of Modern Neuroscience* (New York: McGraw Hill, 2020).
9. S.W. Porges, *The Polyvagal Theory: Neurophysiological Foundations of Emotions, Attachment, Communication, and Self-Regulation* (New York: W.W. Norton, 2011), 267–273; Dana, *Polyvagal Theory in Therapy*, 94–96; Porges, "Polyvagal Perspective," 116–118; A.N. Schore, *The Development of the Unconscious Mind* (New York: W.W. Norton, 2019), 131–135.
10. Daniel J. Siegel, *Mindsight: The New Science of Personal Transformation* (New York: Random House Publishing Group, 2010).
11. J.A. Waxenbaum, V. Reddy, and M. Varacallo, "Anatomy, Autonomic Nervous System" (https://www.ncbi.nlm.nih.gov/books/NBK539845/). 2021 Jul 29. In: *StatPearls* [Internet]. Treasure Island, FL: StatPearls Publishing; 2022 Jan. Accessed 6/15/2023.
12. Chapter 9: Autonomic Nervous System, in E.J. Nestler, P.J. Kenny, S.J. Russo, and A. Schaefer, eds., *Nestler, Hyman & Malenka's Molecular Neuropharmacology: A Foundation for Clinical Neuroscience*, 4th ed. (New York: McGraw Hill, 2020).
13. Daniel J. Siegel, *The Developing Mind: How Relationships and the Brain Interact to Shape Who We Are*, 2nd ed. (New York: Guilford Press, 2012); Annie Wright, "What Is the Window of Tolerance, and Why Is It So Important?," *Psychology Today*, accessed September 10, 2024, https://www.psychologytoday.com/us/blog/trusting-in-relationship/201904/what-is-the-window-of-tolerance-and-why-is-it-so-important.
14. Kathryn Ashton, Alisha R. Davies, Karen Hughes, Kat Ford, Andrew Cotter-Roberts, and Mark A. Bellis, "Adult Support during Childhood: A Retrospective Study of

Trusted Adult Relationships, Sources of Personal Adult Support and Their Association with Childhood Resilience Resources," *BMC Psychology* 9, no. 1 (2021): 101, https://doi .org/10.1186/s40359-021-00601-x.

15. Gerard J. Tortora and Bryan H. Derrickson, *Principles of Anatomy and Physiology* (Hoboken, NJ: Wiley, 2018).
16. Suzanne C. Segerstrom and Gregory E. Miller, "Psychological Stress and the Human Immune System: A Meta-Analytic Study of 30 Years of Inquiry," *Psychological Bulletin* 130, no. 4 (2004): 601–630; Emeran Mayer, *The Mind-Gut Connection: How the Hidden Conversation within Our Bodies Impacts Our Mood, Our Choices, and Our Overall Health* (New York: Harper Wave, 2016); Marilia Carabotti, Annunziata Scirocco, Maria Antonietta Maselli, and Carola Severi, "The Gut-Brain Axis: Interactions between Enteric Microbiota, Central and Enteric NSs," *Annals of Gastroenterology* 28, no. 2 (2015): 203–209.
17. Emeran A. Mayer and Kirsten Tillisch, "The Brain-Gut Axis in Abdominal Pain Syndromes," *Annual Review of Medicine* 62 (2011): 381–396.
18. Babette Rothschild, *The Body Remembers: The Psychophysiology of Trauma and Trauma Treatment* (New York: W.W. Norton, 2000).
19. Porges, *Polyvagal Theory.*
20. James J. Gross and Robert W. Levenson, "Emotional Suppression: Physiology, Self-Report, and Expressive Behavior," *Journal of Personality and Social Psychology* 64, no. 6 (1993): 970–986.
21. Emily A. Butler, Boris Egloff, Frank H. Wilhelm, Nancy C. Smith, Elizabeth A. Erickson, and James J. Gross, "The Social Consequences of Expressive Suppression," *Emotion* 3, no. 1 (2003): 48–67.
22. J.H. Krystal, "Integration and Self-Healing: Affect, Trauma, Alexithymia," *American Journal of Psychiatry* 146, no. 3 (1989): 391–392.
23. Jane M. Richards and James J. Gross, "Emotion Regulation and Memory: The Cognitive Costs of Keeping One's Cool," *Journal of Personality and Social Psychology* 79, no. 3 (2000): 410–424.
24. Richards and Gross, "Emotion Regulation and Memory," 410–424.

Chapter 4: Shame and the Self-Abandonment Cycle

1. Brené Brown, "Shame vs. Guilt," *From Brené* (blog), January 15, 2013, https://brenebrown .com/articles/2013/01/15/shame-v-guilt/.
2. E.J.R. David and Annie O. Derthick, "What Is Internalized Oppression, and So What?," in *The Handbook of Ethical Research with Ethnocultural Populations and Communities*, ed. J.E. Trimble and C.B. Fisher (Thousand Oaks, CA: Sage Publications, 2006), 327–349.
3. Brené Brown, "Shame and Empathy: The Good, the Bad, and the Ugly," *Journal of Counseling and Development* 87, no. 2 (2009): 200–206; June Price Tangney and Ronda L. Dearing, *Shame and Guilt* (New York: Guilford Press, 2002).
4. Michael Lewis, *Shame: The Exposed Self* (New York: Free Press, 1995).
5. W.R.D. Fairbairn, *Psychoanalytic Studies of the Personality* (London: Routledge & Kegan Paul, 1952), 66.
6. Jonathan Caspi, "Sibling Aggression: Assessment and Treatment," in *Sibling Development: Implications for Mental Health Practitioners* (New York: Springer, 2011), 201–219; Kylie Agllias, *Family Scapegoats: Black Sheep and Invisible Children* (London: Routledge, 2018).
7. Sheldon Cohen and Thomas A. Wills, "Stress, Social Support, and the Buffering Hypothesis," *Psychological Bulletin* 98, no. 2 (1985): 310–357.
8. James Prochaska and Carlo DiClemente, *Changing for Good* (New York: William Morrow, 1994), 47.

9. Kristin Neff, *Self-Compassion: The Proven Power of Being Kind to Yourself* (New York: William Morrow, 2011), 24.
10. Brené Brown, *Daring Greatly: How the Courage to Be Vulnerable Transforms the Way We Live, Love, Parent, and Lead* (New York: Gotham Books, 2012); Sue Gerhardt, *Why Love Matters: How Affection Shapes a Baby's Brain* (London: Routledge, 2004); Gabor Maté, *When the Body Says No: Exploring the Stress-Disease Connection* (Hoboken, NJ: Wiley, 2003).
11. Brené Brown, *The Gifts of Imperfection* (Center City, MN: Hazelden Publishing, 2010), 95.
12. Ivan Boszormenyi-Nagy and Barbara Krasner, *Between Give and Take: A Clinical Guide to Contextual Therapy* (New York: Brunner/Mazel, 1986), 102.
13. Neff, *Self-Compassion*, 89.
14. S. Nolen-Hoeksema, B.E. Wisco, and S. Lyubomirsky, "Rethinking Rumination," *Perspectives on Psychological Science* 3, no. 5 (2008): 400–424; A. Aldao, S. Nolen-Hoeksema, and S. Schweizer, "Emotion-Regulation Strategies across Psychopathology: A Meta-analytic Review," *Clinical Psychology Review* 30, no. 2 (2010): 217–237.
15. Jiang, Xiaowei, Huijun Zhang, Xiao Chen, Yanchao Bi, Jing Luo, and Jia Liu, "A Dorsomedial Prefrontal Cortex-Based Dynamic Functional Connectivity Marker for Rumination." *Nature Communications* 14, no. 1 (June 15, 2023): 3431. https://doi.org/10.1038/s41467-023-39142-9.
16. Amir Levine and Rachel Heller, *Attached: The New Science of Adult Attachment and How It Can Help You Find—and Keep—Love* (New York: TarcherPerigee, 2010), 97–98.
17. Martiño Rodríguez-González, Elizabeth A. Skowron, Virginia Cagigal de Gregorio, and Iciar Muñoz San Roque, "Differentiation of Self and Dyadic Adjustment in Couple Relationships: A Scoping Review," *Frontiers in Psychology* 9 (June 2018): 1–13, https://doi.org/10.3389/fpsyg.2018.01133; Elizabeth A. Skowron and Myrna L. Friedlander, "The Differentiation of Self Inventory: Development and Initial Validation," *Journal of Counseling Psychology* 45, no. 3 (July 1998): 235–246; Stephen A. Anderson and Ronald M. Sabatelli, "The Differentiation in the Family System Scale (DIFS)," *American Journal of Family Therapy* 20, no. 1 (1992): 77–89.
18. Erik H. Erikson, *Identity: Youth and Crisis* (New York: W.W. Norton, 1994); Laurence Steinberg, *Adolescence* (New York: McGraw-Hill Education, 2010); Robert Kegan, *In Over Our Heads: The Mental Demands of Modern Life* (Cambridge, MA: Harvard University Press, 1994); Susan Harter, *The Construction of the Self: A Developmental Perspective* (New York: Guilford Press, 1999).
19. Otto F. Kernberg, "Projection and Projective Identification: Developmental and Clinical Aspects," *Journal of the American Psychoanalytic Association* 59, no. 3 (2011): 575–601; Jerome S. Blackman, "Defense Mechanisms: Theoretical, Research and Clinical Perspectives," *Journal of the American Psychoanalytic Association* 53, no. 4 (2005): 1081–1106.
20. Michael S. Levy, "A Helpful Way to Conceptualize and Understand Reenactments," *Journal of Psychotherapy Practice and Research* 7, no. 3 (1998): 227–235, https://www.ncbi.nlm.nih.gov/pmc/articles/PMC3330499/.
21. M.J. Horowitz, *Stress Response Syndrome* (Northvale, NJ: Jason Aronson, 1976); H. Krystal, "Trauma and Affects," *Psychoanalytic Study of the Child* 33 (1978): 81–116; J.L. Herman, *Trauma and Recovery* (New York: Basic Books, 1992); B.A. van der Kolk and A.C. McFarlane, "The Black Hole of Trauma," in *Traumatic Stress: The Effects of Overwhelming Experience on Mind, Body, and Society*, ed. B.A. van der Kolk, A.C. McFarlane, and L. Weisaeth (New York: Guilford, 1996), 3–23.
22. Peter A. Levine, "The Compulsion to Repeat the Trauma: Re-enactment, Revictimization, and Masochism," *Connections and Reflections: The GAINS Quarterly* (2007).

23. B.A. van der Kolk, "The Psychological Consequences of Overwhelming Life Experiences," in *Psychological Trauma*, ed. B.A. van der Kolk (Washington, DC: American Psychiatric Press, 1987), 1–30.

Chapter 5: Be the Cake

1. T. Marchant, J. Jaribu, S. Penfold, M. Tanner, and J.A. Schellenberg, "Measuring Newborn Foot Length to Identify Small Babies in Need of Extra Care: A Cross Sectional Hospital Based Study with Community Follow-up in Tanzania," *BMC Public Health* 10, no. 624 (2010), https://doi.org/10.1186/1471-2458-10-624.
2. Paul Gilbert and Jeremy Miles, "Sensitivity to Social Put-Down: Its Relationship to Perceptions of Social Rank, Shame, Social Anxiety, Depression, Anger and Self-Other Blame," *Personality and Individual Differences* 32, no. 4 (2002): 601–614.
3. Seth G. Disner, Christopher G. Beevers, Emily A.P. Haigh, and Aaron T. Beck, "Neural Mechanisms of the Cognitive Model of Depression," *Nature Reviews Neuroscience* 12, no. 8 (2011): 467–477.
4. Kristin Neff, "What Is Self-Compassion?," Self-Compassion, accessed September 13, 2024, https://self-compassion.org/what-is-self-compassion/.
5. Kristin D. Neff, "Self-Compassion: An Alternative Conceptualization of a Healthy Attitude Toward Oneself," *Self and Identity* 2, no. 2 (2003): 85–101; Richard J. Davidson and William Irwin, "The Functional Neuroanatomy of Emotion and Affective Style," *Trends in Cognitive Sciences* 3, no. 1 (1999): 11–21; Richard J. Davidson and William Irwin, "The Functional Neuroanatomy of Emotion and Affective Style," *Trends in Cognitive Sciences* 3, no. 1 (1999): 11–21.
6. Robert F. Anda, Vincent J. Felitti, J. Douglas Bremner, John D. Walker, Charles Whitfield, Bruce D. Perry, et al., "The Enduring Effects of Abuse and Related Adverse Experiences in Childhood," *European Archives of Psychiatry and Clinical Neuroscience* 256, no. 3 (2006): 174–186; Allan N. Schore, "Effects of a Secure Attachment Relationship on Right Brain Development, Affect Regulation, and Infant Mental Health," *Infant Mental Health Journal* 22, no. 1–2 (2001): 7–66; Vincent J. Felitti, R.F. Anda, D. Nordenberg, D.F. Williamson, A.M. Spitz, V. Edwards, et al., "Relationship of Childhood Abuse and Household Dysfunction to Many of the Leading Causes of Death in Adults," *American Journal of Preventive Medicine* 14, no. 4 (1998): 245–258; Bruce D. Perry and Maia Szalavitz, *The Boy Who Was Raised as a Dog: And Other Stories from a Child Psychiatrist's Notebook—What Traumatized Children Can Teach Us About Loss, Love, and Healing* (New York: Basic Books, 2007); Bessel van der Kolk, *The Body Keeps the Score: Brain, Mind, and Body in the Healing of Trauma* (New York: Viking, 2014).
7. William L. Dunlop and Jessica D. Bannon, "Restorative Narratives: Redemptive and Contaminated Stories of Interpersonal Transgressions and Interpersonal Forgiveness," *Journal of Social and Personal Relationships* 34, no. 3 (2017): 370–394.
8. J.C. Borod, "What Self-Talk Reveals About the Brain," *Scientific American*, August 1, 2017, https://www.scientificamerican.com/article/what-self-talk-reveals-about-the-brain/; K.R. Fox, T.E. Johnson, and C.D. Heinen, "Navigating the Landscape of Self-Talk: A Grounded Theory Exploration of Intrapersonal Communication Patterns in the Context of Ultramarathon Running," *Frontiers in Psychology* 14 (2023): 1210960, https://www.frontiersin.org/articles/10.3389/fpsyg.2023.1210960/full; J.J. Hamson-Utley and C.F. Martin, "The Effects of Self-Talk on the Volleyball Serve Performance of Collegiate Women," *Journal of Applied Sport Psychology* 24, no. 4 (2012): 356–365, https://www.ncbi.nlm.nih.gov/pmc/articles/PMC5986836/; D. Roberson, J.R. DeSanto, and T. Morris, "Exploring

Factors Influencing the Language of Self-Talk and Their Potential Impact on Athletic Performance," *Journal of Sport and Exercise Psychology* 43, no. 1 (2021): 42–51, https://www.ncbi.nlm.nih.gov/pmc/articles/PMC8295361/.

9. Lucia Capacchione, *Recovery of Your Inner Child: The Highly Acclaimed Method for Liberating Your Inner Self* (New York: Simon & Schuster, 1991).

Chapter 6: Somatics 101

1. Walter Mignolo, professor of semiotics and literary studies at Duke University, in conversation with the author, December 2022.
2. Laurence J. Kirmayer, Gregory M. Brass, and Caroline L. Tait, "The Mental Health of Aboriginal Peoples: Transformations of Identity and Community," *Canadian Journal of Psychiatry* 45, no. 7 (2000): 607–616; Lewis Mehl-Madrona, "What Traditional Indigenous Elders Say About Cross-Cultural Mental Health Training," *Explore: The Journal of Science and Healing* 6, no. 1 (2010): 38–45; Eduardo Duran, Bonnie Duran, Maria Yellow Horse Brave Heart, and Susan Yellow Horse-Davis, "Healing the American Indian Soul Wound," in *International Handbook of Multigenerational Legacies of Trauma*, ed. Yael Danieli, 341–354 (New York: Plenum Press, 1998); Gregory Cajete, *Native Science: Natural Laws of Interdependence* (Santa Fe, NM: Clear Light Publishers, 2000); Judy Atkinson, *Trauma Trails, Recreating Song Lines: The Transgenerational Effects of Trauma in Indigenous Australia* (North Melbourne: Spinifex Press, 2002); Karina L. Walters and Jane M. Simoni, "Reconceptualizing Native Women's Health: An 'Indigenist' Stress-Coping Model," *American Journal of Public Health* 92, no. 4 (2002): 520–524; Joseph P. Gone, "'We Never Was Happy Living Like a Whiteman': Mental Health Disparities and the Postcolonial Predicament in American Indian Communities," *American Journal of Community Psychology* 40, no. 3–4 (2007): 290–300.
3. Hugo D. Critchley and Sarah N. Garfinkel, "Interactions between Visceral and Cognitive Neural Systems," *Annals of the New York Academy of Sciences* 1351, no. 1 (2015): 58.
4. Peter Payne, Peter A. Levine, and Mardi A. Crane-Godreau, "Somatic Experiencing: Using Interoception and Proprioception as Core Elements of Trauma Therapy," *Frontiers in Psychology* 6 (2015): 93; Emma Brooks, Jessica Flores, Madison Loeser, Alli Nickel, and Hannah Richason, "Healing the Body and Mind: Sensory and Somatic Interventions for Interpersonal Trauma," *Indiana University School of Health and Human Sciences* (2020).
5. Wolf E. Mehling, Cynthia Price, John Daubenmier, Erik Acree, Susan Bartmess, and Anita Stewart, "The Multidimensional Assessment of Interoceptive Awareness (MAIA)," *PLOS ONE* 7, no. 11 (2012): e48230.
6. Marie Kuhfuß, Tobias Maldei, Andreas Hetmanek, and Nicola Baumann, "Somatic Experiencing—Effectiveness and Key Factors of a Body-Oriented Trauma Therapy: A Scoping Literature Review," *European Journal of Psychotraumatology* 12, no. 1 (2021): 1929023.
7. Stephen W. Porges, *The Polyvagal Theory: Neurophysiological Foundations of Emotions, Attachment, Communication, and Self-Regulation*, 1st ed. Norton Series on Interpersonal Neurobiology (New York: W.W. Norton, 2011).
8. R. Hyman, P. Bertelson, M.K. Holland, G.R. Lockhead, R.W. Schvaneveldt, W.G. Chase, et al., "Perceiving Patterns in Random Series: Dynamic Processing of Sequence in Prefrontal Cortex," *Nature Neuroscience*, accessed January 2, 2024, https://www.nature.com/articles/nn0400_282; A.W. MacDonald, J.D. Cohen, V.A. Stenger, C.S. Carter, T.S. Braver, J.D. Cohen, et al., "The Role of Prefrontal Cortex in Cognitive Control and

Executive Function," *Neuropsychopharmacology* (2020), accessed January 2, 2024, https://www.nature.com/articles/s41386-020-00886-7.

9. Hyman et al., "Perceiving Patterns"; MacDonald et al., "Role of Prefrontal Cortex."
10. Cleveland Clinic, "Phrenic Nerve: Anatomy and Function," last reviewed January 9, 2022, accessed January 2, 2024, https://my.clevelandclinic.org/health/body/22270-phrenic-nerve.
11. Kathy L. Kain and Stephen J. Terrell, *Nurturing Resilience: Helping Clients Move Forward from Developmental Trauma—An Integrative Somatic Approach* (Berkeley: North Atlantic Books, 2018).
12. Matthew McKay, Jeffrey C. Wood, and Jeffrey Brantley, *The Dialectical Behavior Therapy Skills Workbook: Practical DBT Exercises for Learning Mindfulness, Interpersonal Effectiveness, Emotion Regulation, and Distress Tolerance* (Oakland CA: New Harbinger Publications, 2007).
13. Sigrid Breit, Aleksandra Kupferberg, Gerhard Rogler, and Gregor Hasler, "Vagus Nerve as Modulator of the Brain–Gut Axis in Psychiatric and Inflammatory Disorders," *Frontiers in Psychiatry* 9 (2018): 44, https://doi.org/10.3389/fpsyt.2018.00044; Andrea Zaccaro, Andrea Piarulli, Marco Laurino, Erika Garbella, Danilo Menicucci, Bruno Neri, et al., "How Breath-Control Can Change Your Life: A Systematic Review on Psycho-Physiological Correlates of Slow Breathing," *Frontiers in Human Neuroscience* 12 (2018): 353, https://doi.org/10.3389/fnhum.2018.00353.
14. Babette Rothschild, *The Body Remembers: The Psychophysiology of Trauma and Trauma Treatment* (New York: W.W. Norton, 2000); Porges, *Polyvagal Theory.*
15. Noa Belling, *The Mindful Body: Build Emotional Strength and Manage Stress with Body Mindfulness* (Sydney: Rockpool Publishing, 2018).
16. Carl R. Rogers, *Client-Centered Therapy: Its Current Practice, Implications, and Theory* (Boston: Houghton Mifflin, 1951).
17. Sigal Zilcha-Mano, Mario Mikulincer, and Phillip R. Shaver, "Pet in the Therapy Room: An Attachment Perspective on Animal-Assisted Therapy," *Attachment and Human Development* 13, no. 6 (2011): 541–561.
18. Stephen W. Porges, *The Pocket Guide to the Polyvagal Theory: The Transformative Power of Feeling Safe*, 1st ed. Norton Series on Interpersonal Neurobiology (New York: W.W. Norton, 2017).
19. Deb Dana, *The Polyvagal Theory in Therapy: Engaging the Rhythm of Regulation* (New York: W.W. Norton, 2018).
20. M. Noetel, T. Sanders, D. Gallardo-Gómez, P. Taylor, B. del Pozo Cruz, D. van den Hoek, et al., "Effect of Exercise for Depression: Systematic Review and Network Meta-analysis of Randomised Controlled Trials," *BMJ* 384 (2024): e075847, https://doi.org/10.1136/bmj-2023-075847.
21. Robin L. Carhart-Harris, David Erritzoe, Tim Williams, James M. Stone, Laurence J. Reed, Alessandro Colasanti, et al., "Neural Correlates of the Psychedelic State as Determined by fMRI Studies with Psilocybin," *Proceedings of the National Academy of Sciences* 109, no. 6 (2012): 2138–2143.

Chapter 7: The Thought Work Protocol

1. Viktor E. Frankl, *Man's Search for Meaning*, trans. Ilse Lasch (Boston: Beacon Press, 2006).
2. Karen Lawson, "What Are Thoughts and Emotions?," Taking Charge of Your Wellbeing, University of Minnesota, https://www.takingcharge.csh.umn.edu/what-are-thoughts

-emotions. Accessed 8/2/2023; Carroll E. Izard, "Emotion Theory and Research: Highlights, Unanswered Questions, and Emerging Issues," *Annual Review of Psychology* 60, no. 1 (2009): 1–25.

3. Daniel J. Siegel, *Mindsight: The New Science of Personal Transformation* (New York: Random House Publishing Group, 2010).
4. Inger Sundström-Poromaa, and Erika Gingnell, "Menstrual Cycle Influence on Cognitive Function and Emotion Processing—From a Reproductive Perspective," *Frontiers in Neuroscience* 8, no. 380 (2014), https://doi.org/10.3389/fnins.2014.00380; J. Bayer, J. Rune, and O. Hausmann, "The Cycling Brain: Menstrual Cycle Related Fluctuations in Cognition and Emotion in Women," *Neuroscience & Biobehavioral Reviews* 115 (2020): 180–202, https://doi.org/10.1016/j.neubiorev.2020.05.002; Kimberly A. Yonkers et al., "Premenstrual Syndrome," *StatPearls*, 2023, https://www.ncbi.nlm.nih.gov/books/NBK560698/, accessed 8/14/2023.
5. John E. Sarno, *Healing Back Pain: The Mind-Body Connection* (New York: Warner Books, 1991).
6. Nicole Sachs, *The Meaning of Truth: Embrace Your Truth, Create Your Life* (pub. by author, 2016).

Chapter 8: Boundaries, Limits, and Direct Communication

1. Henry Cloud and John Sims Townsend, *Boundaries: When to Say Yes, When to Say No to Take Control of Your Life* (Grand Rapids, MI: Zondervan Publishing House, 2012).
2. Anne Katherine, *Where to Draw the Line: How to Set Healthy Boundaries Every Day* (New York: Simon & Schuster, 2000).
3. John Sims Townsend, *Beyond Boundaries: Learning to Trust Again in Relationships* (Waterville, ME: Christian Large Print, 2012).

Index

ABOUT THE AUTHOR

Beatriz Victoria Albina, is a UCSF-trained nurse practitioner, master-certified somatic life coach, and somatic experiencing practitioner with a master's in public health. A proud Oberlin College grad (class of flannel shirts and Ani DiFranco on repeat), she is the creator of the term Emotional Outsourcing™—her verbiage for the codependent, perfectionist, and people-pleasing thought habits that disconnect people from their self-trust, boundaries, and authentic desires.

Béa (Bay-ah) is known for her compassionate, sharp, science-backed approach that bridges nervous system regulation, somatic healing, and intersectional feminism. Her work unpacks how childhood emotional conditioning, socialization, and systems of oppression shape our inner narratives—and how reclaiming our bodies as safe homes can change everything.

Through her flagship program *Anchored*, her podcast *Feminist Wellness*, and her courses in nervous system education and somatics, she's helped thousands of smart, self-aware folks finally stop performing for love and start living in alignment with their values. Her work is both deeply educational and radically tender, rooted in the belief that you don't have to earn your worth—you're already worthy of being met, held, and known, without the performance, without the pretending, without tap-dancing for your lovability.

Born in Mar del Plata, Argentina, Béa grew up in the great state of Rhode Island. She lives in New York with her wife, Billey, a mischievous cat named Wade, and a deep reverence for the earth beneath her feet.

SUBSCRIBE TO THE *FEMINIST WELLNESS* PODCAST!

This book grew out of my podcast, *Feminist Wellness*, where I've spent years unpacking the science of healing, the psychology of Emotional Outsourcing, and the somatics of self-trust through an intersectional feminist lens—all with a hefty dose of warmth, wit, plenty of silly pet names, and zero tolerance for snake oil (#BecauseScience). There are *hundreds* of episodes waiting for you, packed with free, in-depth explorations of nervous system regulation, attachment, boundaries, and what it actually takes to stop outsourcing your worth to overcome those sneaky ol' codependent, perfectionist, and people-pleasing habits. It's wellness without the fluff: all the science, all the woo, none of the nonsense.

And if you find yourself wanting more—more nuance, more depth, more of the threads I couldn't fully weave together here because a book can only have so many pages—the podcast is where you'll find it. It's absolutely free and I can't wait to share it with you.

Scan the QR code below to be directed to the show—subscribe/follow wherever you get your podcasts and dive into the archive—you'll find a treasure trove of insights to support your healing.

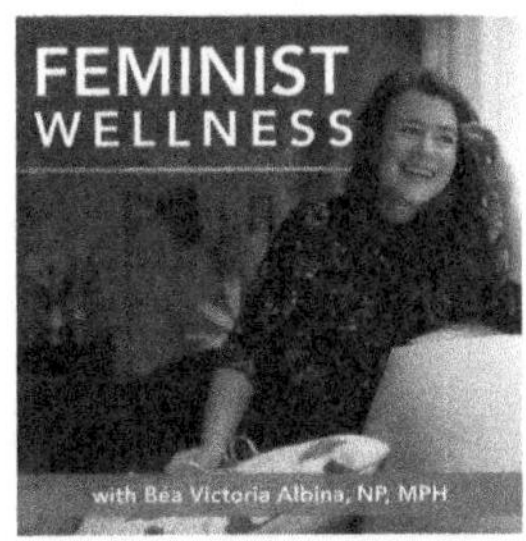

RAISING READERS

Books Build Bright Futures

Thank you for reading this book and for being a reader of books in general. As an author, I am so grateful to share being part of a community of readers with you, and I hope you will join me in passing our love of books on to the next generation of readers.

Did you know that reading for enjoyment is the single biggest predictor of a child's future happiness and success?

More than family circumstances, parents' educational background, or income, reading impacts a child's future academic performance, emotional well-being, communication skills, economic security, ambition, and happiness.

Studies show that kids reading for enjoyment in the US is in rapid decline:

- In 2012, 53% of 9-year-olds read almost every day. Just 10 years later, in 2022, the number had fallen to 39%.
- In 2012, 27% of 13-year-olds read for fun daily. By 2023, that number was just 14%.

Together, we can commit to **Raising Readers** and change this trend. How?

- Read to children in your life daily.
- Model reading as a fun activity.
- Reduce screen time.
- Start a family, school, or community book club.
- Visit bookstores and libraries regularly.
- Listen to audiobooks.
- Read the book before you see the movie.
- Encourage your child to read aloud to a pet or stuffed animal.
- Give books as gifts.
- Donate books to families and communities in need.

BOB1217

Books build bright futures, and **Raising Readers** is our shared responsibility.

For more information, visit **JoinRaisingReaders.com**

Sources: National Endowment for the Arts, National Assessment of Educational Progress, WorldBookDay.org, Nielsen BookData's 2023 "Understanding the Children's Book Consumer"